OXFORD MEDICAL PUBL

CW01461016

Textbook of Rehabilitation Medicine

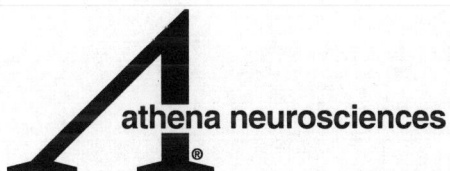

Textbook of Rehabilitation Medicine

....

Michael P. Barnes
Professor of Neurological Rehabilitation,
University of Newcastle upon Tyne, Hunters Moor Regional
Rehabilitation Centre, Newcastle upon Tyne, UK

and

Anthony B. Ward
Consultant/Senior Lecturer in Rehabilitation Medicine,
North Staffordshire Rehabilitation Centre,
Stoke on Trent, UK

OXFORD
UNIVERSITY PRESS

OXFORD

UNIVERSITY PRESS

Great Clarendon Street, Oxford OX2 6DP

Oxford University Press is a department of the University of Oxford.
It furthers the University's objectives of excellence in research, scholarship,
and education by publishing worldwide in

Oxford New York

Athens Auckland Bangkok Bogotá Buenos Aires Calcutta
Cape Town Chennai Dar es Salaam Delhi Florence Hong Kong Istanbul
Karachi Kuala Lumpur Madrid Melbourne Mexico City Mumbai
Nairobi Paris São Paulo Singapore Taipei Tokyo Toronto Warsaw

and associated companies in Berlin Ibadan

Oxford is a registered trade mark of Oxford University Press
in the UK and in certain other countries

Published in the United States
by Oxford University Press, Inc., New York

British Library Cataloguing in Publication Data
Data available

Library of Congress Cataloging in Publication Data

Barnes, Michael, MD, FRCP.
Textbook of rehabilitation medicine / Michael P. Barnes and Anthony B. Ward
p. ; cm. — (Oxford medical publications)
Includes bibliographical references and index.
1. Medical rehabilitation. I. Ward, Anthony B. II. Title. III. Series.
[DNLM: 1. Rehabilitation. WB 320 B26lt 2000]
RM930 B37 2000   617'.03—dc21   99-046510

1 3 5 7 9 10 8 6 4 2

ISBN 0 19 262805 4

Typset by Downdell, Oxford
Printed in Great Britain
on acid-free paper by
Biddles Ltd,
Guildford & King's Lynn

Contents

....

Section A

General principles of rehabilitation

1

···

Concepts of rehabilitation

Rehabilitation is rather different from other medical specialities. It is a process that is based on the principles of education and one in which the disabled person and their family must be involved for it to have any meaning. It is also a process that has to go beyond the narrow confines of physical disease and must also deal with the psychological consequences of physical disability and with the social milieu in which the disabled person has to operate. Herein is another dimension which differentiates rehabilitation from most of medicine—it is a process that cannot be carried out by physicians alone and requires active partnership with a range of other health and social service professionals. It is essentially a team process in which the doctor clearly has an important role to play but a role that is not always paramount.

Modern rehabilitation practice is based around the concepts of impairment, disability, and handicap as outlined by the World Health Organization in 1980 (Table 1.1).

Impairment is a descriptive term. It says nothing about consequence. A left hemiparesis or bi-temporal hemianopia are descriptions of impairments. These descriptions are essential parts of a diagnostic process but otherwise are of limited value. Rehabilitation goes beyond impairment and places impairments within their functional context—the

Table 1.1 Definitions of the WHO's International Classification of Impairments, Disabilities, and Handicaps (1980).

Impairment	Any loss or abnormality of psychological, physiological or anatomical structure or function
Disability	Any restriction or lack of activity resulting from an impairment to perform an activity in the manner or in the range considered normal for people of the same age, sex and culture.
Handicap	A disadvantage for a given individual resulting from impairment or disability that limits or prevents the fulfilment of a role that would otherwise be normal for that individual.

disability. There is not necessarily a clear hierarchical relationship between impairment and the consequent disability. For example, a left hemiparesis (the impairment) can lead to a complete inability to walk, the ability to walk only with the aid of a stick or the ability to walk independently but with some difficulty over, for instance, rough ground. Thus, the impairment can result in a number of different disabilities. It is the disability that matters to the individual and not the impairment.

Handicap describes the social context of the disability. For example, inability to walk over rough ground may be a major problem for a gardener and indeed may preclude employment. However, for an older person living in a nursing home such a disability may present no handicap and offer no limitation to a desired lifestyle. Rehabilitation is largely concerned with disability and handicap.

Rehabilitation can thus be defined as an active and dynamic process by which a disabled person is helped to acquire knowledge and skills in order to maximize physical, psychological, and social function. It is a process that maximizes functional ability and minimizes disability and handicap. An understanding of this process is important as it allows conceptionalization of the three basic rehabilitation approaches:

• approaches to reduce disability

- approaches designed to acquire new skills and strategies which will reduce the impact of disability
- approaches that help to alter the environment, both the physical environment and the social environment, so that a given disability carries with it as little handicap as possible.

Take an example of a middle-aged man with multiple sclerosis who is married with two children and is still working as an accounts clerk. He is developing increasing problems walking, mainly secondary to spasticity, as well as difficulties with urinary frequency, urgency, and occasional incontinence. Rehabilitation in this example could be directed towards:

1. Measures to reduce his disability by attention to spasticity and medication to help control his bladder symptoms.
2. He could learn new skills such as walking with support or perhaps using a wheelchair for longer distances in order to minimize fatigue.
3. He could learn to adjust his regime at work and socially in order to allow regular access to a toilet and may need to learn new skills such as intermittent self-catheterization.
4. Another approach may be to adapt his environment both at home and work to make it easier for him to manage. There may be a need for grab rails in the toilet and adaptations to the bathroom or kitchen. Liaison with his employers may be important to make similar physical adaptations to his work. He may wish to negotiate with his employers to work part-time or allow him a few short rest breaks during the day to minimize his fatigue. It may be appropriate to work with his wife and children in order to involve them more in acceptance of his deteriorating condition and adjustment to their own lifestyle.

A whole range of other options may be appropriate within all three areas. The beauty of rehabilitation often comes from helping the disabled person and family to see new ways of developing skills, new strategies, and new approaches to life with the fundamental aim of maximizing quality of life.

Terminology

Rehabilitation is an individual, active, and dynamic process. It is important to avoid terminology that implies dependency or terminology which simply serves to categorize all disabled people. The word patient is entirely appropriate for someone who is acutely ill and dependent upon medical and health professionals. It is not a term that is appropriate for a disabled individual striving towards independence and the development of new skills. The term client, commonly used within social services, has implications of a business and contractual relationship which is also inappropriate in a health setting. There is actually no adequate word in the English language that describes the relationship between the rehabilitation team and disabled person. Other group classifications are also unnecessary and terms such as 'epileptics', 'stroke sufferers', 'spastics', or even 'the disabled' are entirely inappropriate. This is not simply political correctness. Terminology can be insulting and demeaning but more importantly indicates an inappropriate philosophy and an inappropriate attitude and approach to disabled people.

Medical and social models of disability

For a number of years there have been two philosophically opposed camps within the field of disability. The so-called 'medical model of disability' can be characterized by the disabled person taking or being forced into a dependent and passive position and having goals and strategies imposed on them by the rehabilitation team. It is an autocratic, 'we know best' system which may be caring but does nothing to promote independence, enablement, and self-esteem. The so-called 'social model of disability' has roots in the United States and developed from the attitudes and beliefs of disabled veterans from the Vietnam War. The social model places much more emphasis on the faults of society. The view is that society is not sufficiently adjusted and attuned to the needs of the disabled person, not just in terms of physical accessibility but in terms of a cultural attitude that makes it difficult to accept deviations from the norm. This is a simplistic and somewhat polarized overview of the two apparently opposed models. It can be summarized as one model focusing on the disabled person as having a problem and the other focusing on society having a problem. However, few individuals or organizations adopt either of these views in their entirety. Many people are now working towards a partnership model of disability that does recognize the value and contribution that can be made by a rehabilitation team, particularly in the post-acute stages after trauma, whilst at the same time recognizing that longer-term disability can and should be alleviated by societal attitudinal change and backed up with appropriate anti-discrimination legislation. In recognition of the importance of the influence of society the World Health Organization is currently piloting a new classification system. The new suggested classification (International Classification of Impairments, Disabilities and Handicaps—2) replaces the term Disabilities by Activities and replaces Handicap by Participation. The emphasis of classification is now more positive—emphasizing individual abilities and a role in society rather than the somewhat negative concepts of disabilities and handicap. It is hoped that this new classification will meet the need for an international common language for the consequence of diseases and other health conditions and provide users with operational tools for measurement and comparison. The new system includes a classification of contextual factors—environmental and personal factors that modulate the experience of disablement for individuals. The new classification is currently undergoing evaluation and should be revised and fully adopted in the near future.

The process of rehabilitation

The basic nature of rehabilitation is to work with the disabled person and family in partnership. The professionals should impart accurate information and advice, give guidance on prognosis and natural history, and help the individual establish realistic goals within an appropriate social context. The team should then use their professional expertise to implement treatment and management programmes designed to fulfil the goals set by the disabled person. Some individuals will want to take a major leading role in developing their own goals whilst others will wish to take a more passive role and rely on the expertise of the team. Some families and carers will want to have a say or even act as advocates for the disabled person, particularly if there are cognitive and intellectual problems. Clearly there is room for conflict between the team's view of a realistic goal, the disabled person's view and the carer's view. Such conflicts will need to be resolved, sometimes by reference to an external advocate, but usually by a process of discussion and negotiation. If rehabilitation is to be taken forward, agreed goals and outcomes are essential. In some units a written, informal contract has been used as a way of making mutual responsibilities clear. However, it is important to emphasize that a rehabilitation team must be prepared to have its thoughts and suggestions criticized not only by other team members but by the disabled person and family. It is sometimes necessary for the team to work towards goals which they do not see themselves to be priorities but are seen to be important by that individual.

Thus the essence of rehabilitation is goal setting. The first goal is a long-distance strategic aim. This can vary enormously. In an individual after stroke the aim may be a return to a completely normal pre-stroke lifestyle. For others, with the likelihood of residual disabilities or for those with deteriorating conditions, the long-term strategic goal will need to be set at a different level. A goal for someone with a severe head injury may simply be to return to home and remain at home with the help of formal or informal carers. It may be to take up part-time employment or resume a particular previous leisure interest. The overall strategic goal can obviously have a number of long-term sub-goals relating to different spheres of life such as employment, home, and leisure.

The goal setting should be a dynamic process that can be changed and adjusted according to progress.

After the long-term goal steps will need to be defined in order to achieve that goal. If, for example, the long-term goal is independent walking then achievement of that will require a breakdown into a number of shorter-term goals such as sitting without support, standing without support, walking with assistance, walking with aids, and finally independent walking. A short-term goal should always have a number of key criteria. These are usefully remembered by the mnemonic SMART. Goals should be:

Specific
Measurable
Achievable
Relevant
Time-limited

Specific goals are precise. An inappropriate goal would be 'to walk with an improved gait'. This is not sufficiently specific nor is it readily measurable. A more specific and measurable goal would be to walk 20 metres with the aid of a stick within 30 seconds. Such specificity and measurability is essential in order to avoid descent into a vague and unfocused programme. The goals should clearly be achievable within a specified time frame which should preferably be reasonably short. If a time frame is denoted in months then progress is difficult to monitor with accuracy. It is better to break down such goals into more achievable weekly or fortnightly steps. Finally the goals should be desired by that person and relevant to that person's social context. It may be better for a young man to have a goal of opening a can of lager rather than making a cup of tea!

Outcome measurement

The implication of goal setting is that the team and disabled person should know when the goals have been achieved. Valid and reliable outcome measures are thus important tools to be used by the rehabilitation team. There are a number of specific outcome measures that can monitor overall disability and handicap as well as more specific outcomes for specific functions such as

mobility, hand function, or various psychological parameters such as memory. This subject is covered in more
detail in Chapter 5.

Benefits of rehabilitation

What are the benefits that can follow from a proper
rehabilitation process?

Functional benefit

Some of the benefit of rehabilitation is obvious. The supply
of a wheelchair, for example, to someone who is unable to
walk is an immediate and self-evident benefit. However, at
a broader level is there evidence that a coordinated interdisciplinary rehabilitation approach can produce a better
functional outcome for an individual over more traditional
service delivery? There is now documentation that this is
the case. There is clear evidence, particularly from the
literature on stroke rehabilitation, of functional gain and
improved outcome. Individuals who have gone through a
stroke rehabilitation unit stand a higher chance of return-
ing to their own homes and less risk of living within an
institutional, nursing, or residential home environment. In
addition to improved function the individuals also tend to
obtain their final functional level more quickly than in a
less focused environment. However, there is also evidence
that such functional gains are lost if rehabilitation does not
continue after discharge. In one study, people with stroke
were better off at discharge from a rehabilitation unit than
those who had been managed in a general medical ward
but at one year, without rehabilitation follow-up, the
benefits had been lost and the two groups were functionally similar. Short-term post-acute rehabilitation must be
followed by longer-term support and follow-up. There is
also evidence of similar gains following rehabilitation for
people with spinal cord injuries, head injuries, and even in
deteriorating conditions such as multiple sclerosis. Coordinated input will not only reduce physical problems but
there is also evidence of psychological benefit. There is

evidence of less depression and anxiety and better function, through coping strategies, of cognitive and intellectual problems. Carers feel better supported and have fewer psychological problems. There is better delivery of information and more knowledge of the disease process amongst those with access to a rehabilitation team. Overall the disabled person and family prefer the rehabilitation setting than more traditional hospital care.

Reduction in unnecessary complications

Related to functional gain is the avoidance of unnecessary disability and handicap. A number of problems are preventable such as contractures, pressure sores, and untreated depression. A rehabilitation team should be able to monitor the individual and prevent such unnecessary complications arising.

Coordination and better use of resources

A person, particularly with complex and severe disabilities, will need a variety of health, social, and other services. These services need coordination to prevent unnecessary overlap of assessment and treatment. A rehabilitation team should be in a better position to coordinate such services and act as a single point of contact for the disabled person and family. The team should be in a better position to liaise with a wide network of necessary support services and develop personal contacts in fields as diverse as employment, education, and housing. Such a network, properly applied and coordinated, should lead to a better chance of minimizing handicap.

Cost effective

At the present time there are very few studies that analyse the health economics of a rehabilitation team. However, it seems likely that prevention of unnecessary duplication of assessment and treatment and better coordination as well as functional gains and unnecessary longer-term complications should all mean that access to a rehabilitation team will be cost effective. Unnecessary crisis admissions should be avoided, as problems should be predicted. In broader economic terms, if the disabled person can be assisted back to work, even on a part-time basis, this will be a major cost saving for the national economy. About 80 per cent of the costs for disability are due to lost employment opportunities.

Education, training, and research

There is a pressing need for education and training both of the rehabilitation team and the wider network of health and social service professionals in disability issues. A rehabilitation team could and should act as a focus for education and training for themselves and others as well as for disabled people. A team, particularly in an academic setting, should also act as a focus for rehabilitation research which is badly needed in order to place rehabilitation on a proper evidence-based foundation.

Conclusions

This chapter has outlined the concepts, principles, and process of rehabilitation and some of the benefits that can follow. Rehabilitation is essentially a process of education and enablement that intrinsically involves the disabled person and his or her family. It is a process that is conducted through a series of specific goals as a route to a long-term strategic aim. The process can produce real benefit in terms of function, fewer unnecessary complications, better coordination, cost effectiveness, and general education of health professionals and disabled people in the wide field of disability. Rehabilitation is often thought to be a vague and woolly process, and indeed in the past this has often been the case. Modern rehabilitation is a combination of a precise science and the art of traditional medicine. It should be a rewarding process, both for the professional and the disabled person.

Further reading

Barnes, M. P. and Oliver, M. (1993). Organization of neurological rehabilitation services. In: Greenwood, R., Barnes, M. P., McMillan, T. M., and Ward, C. D. (ed.) *Neurological rehabilitation*, pp.29–40. Churchill Livingstone, London.

Dobkin, B. H. (ed.) (1996). *Neurologic rehabilitation*. Davis, Philadelphia.

Glanville, H. J. (1994). What is rehabilitation? In: Illis, L. S. (ed.) *Neurological rehabilitation* (2nd edn), pp.7–13. Blackwell Scientific, London.

Good, D. C. and Couch, J. R. (1994). *Handbook of neurorehabilitation. Part II—Outcome measures and the rehabilitation process*, pp.105–77. Marcel Dekker, New York.

Lazar, R. B. (1998). *Principles of neurologic rehabilitation*. McGraw-Hill, New York.

Wade, D. T. (1996). *Measurement in neurological rehabilitation*. Oxford University Press, Oxford.

World Health Organization.(1998). *The world health report—1998. Life in the 21st century—a vision for ALL*. WHO, Geneva. (A useful reference on a number of world health issues but in particular includes a discussion of the new classification of impairments, activities, and participation.)

2

....

Epidemiology

Epidemiology is the study of patterns of disease occurrence in populations and of factors that influence these patterns. It may seem strange to discuss this early in the book, but such discussion puts the whole issue of disability into perspective, and allows us to put individual conditions into perspective. Knowledge of epidemiology is linked with the natural history of a disease or condition, and is therefore relevant to clinical practice.

Incidence and prevalence

The incidence of a condition is defined as the number of new cases appearing in a unit time, such as a year. The prevalence refers to the number of people in the community affected by their condition at any one time and the differences between the two may be small or large depending on the survival of patients. Non-progressive disorders in young people, for instance, can have a very high prevalence and therefore a significant impact on the allocation of resources. This typifies the situation in osteoarthritis, stroke, traumatic brain injury, etc., whereas rapidly progressive problems such as cancers and motor neurone disease require rapid flexible responses in the knowledge that service provision may require change after only a short time. This approach is at present not well catered for by rehabilitation services. In contrast to acute medical services, the planning of disability services is more concerned with prevalence than with incidence. The Office of Population Census and Surveys (OPCS) surveys of disability in Great Britain reported in 1988 and 1989 and contributed greatly to the knowledge of disability in the UK It recognized six million disabled people in the UK and devised a weighting system to provide a severity grade of 1 (least severe) to 10 (most severe). It also identified thirteen domains of disability, based on the ICIDH criteria, which are set out in Table 2.1.

The OPCS survey found that the prevalence of disability among adults was 135 per 1000 population, aged 16 years and over. If one includes those people living in institu-

Table 2.1   Disability domains—estimates of prevalence of disability in Great Britain by type (ICIDH) and age per 1000 population. (Source: Martin, Meltzer, and Elliott 1988.)

Type of disability	Age group			
	16–59	60–74	75+	All adults
Locomotion	31	198	496	99
Hearing	17	110	328	59
Personal care	18	99	313	57
Dexterity	13	78	199	40
Seeing	9	56	262	38
Intellectual function	20	40	109	34
Behaviour	19	40	152	31
Reaching and stretching	9	54	149	28
Communication	12	42	140	27
Continence	9	42	147	26
Disfigurement	5	18	27	9
Eating, drinking, and digesting	2	12	30	6
Consciousness	5	10	9	5

tions, the prevalence increases to 142 per 1000. Table 2.1 identifies the prevalence of each of the thirteen different types, according to age and over three-quarters of disabled people (77 per cent) were found to have one or more of these physical disabilities, implying a prevalence rate of 104.1 per 1000 aged 16 years and over, living in the community, and 109 per 1000, including those living in institutions.

Difficulty with locomotion is the most common disability and has the highest prevalence for all age groups. Physical disability is likely to occur in combination with other types of disability, especially sensory disabilities. The combination of physical and mental disabilities, appears to be the most disabling, as is seen in Table 2.2.

In the United Kingdom most disability is due to musculo-skeletal disease and is followed by problems related to the eye and ear. Generally speaking, neurological conditions make up a smaller component, but have far greater relevance in the more severe categories of disability on the OPCS scale. In fact, severe disability in younger people is primarily due to neurological disease. Table 2.3 gives the frequency of disease groups for adults and private households (OPCS survey).

Severe disability is also associated with multiple pathologies and such people over the age of 60 years are more

Table 2.2 Types of disability by severity category expressed as a percentage within each severity group. (Source: Martin, White, and Meltzer 1989.)

Type of disability	Severity (%)					
	1–2	3–4	5–6	7–8	9–10	Total
Other disability (not physical)	38	26	17	5	0	23
Physical	39	35	31	25	18	33
Physical and sensory	21	31	30	36	28	28
Physical and mental (± sensory)	2	8	24	34	56	18
Total	100	100	100	100	100	100

Table 2.3 Frequency of disease groups causing physical disabilities and all disability—adults in private households (per 1000 population). (Source: Martin, White, and Meltzer 1989, OPCS.)

Disease (ICD group)	All types	Locomotor	Type of disability Reaching and stretching	Dexterity	Disfigurement
Musculoskeletal	46	56	64	67	61
Ear	38	1	0	0	1
Eye	22	2	0	1	2
Circulatory	20	23	10	7	5
Mental	13	3	2	3	1
Nervous system	13	12	21	22	12
Respiratory	13	14	3	2	1
Digestive	6	2	2	1	5
Genitourinary	3	1	1	0	2
Neoplasms	2	1	3	2	4
Endocrine	2	2	1	1	1
Infections	1	1	1	1	3
Blood	1	0	0	0	0
Skin	1	1	0	0	4
Congenital	0	0	0	0	3
Other	6	5	3	4	1

likely to have two or more conditions, which increase with age. Arthritis and hypertension, the two conditions with the highest prevalence, coexisted in more than one-quarter of those aged 60 years and over. Work has shown that, as the number of chronic conditions experienced by older people rises, the prevalence of disability rises almost exponentially. Rehabilitation of older people therefore is much more likely to be associated with comorbid disease and this is one of the essential differences between the rehabilitation of older and younger groups. It is also known that certain conditions are more prevalent in different parts of the country and the classic example is the increase in multiple sclerosis as one moves north throughout Britain. Therefore, services have to reflect the needs of local populations, particularly those for the more common disabling conditions. In addition, the affluence and social circumstances of certain parts of the United Kingdom appears to be reflected by a concomitant change in the levels of disability and disadvantage and this is perhaps based on occupational and different levels of educational attainment and income.

How does epidemiological information help us?

Why is it so important to have a good knowledge of epidemiology in order to practice rehabilitation medicine? Firstly, it is important to know whether one is trying to change the impairment, the activity/disability, or the participation/handicap. For instance, if the goal of rehabilitation is to allow a person with impaired mobility to get upstairs and use the bathroom, one could approach the problem in three ways. Firstly, definitive treatment could be directed at the pathology and impairment to diminish their effects and restore function in the limbs. Secondly, the disability could be addressed, with the result that, despite a continuing impairment, the person could be trained to climb the stairs and walk to the bathroom, or thirdly, a chair lift and a wheelchair could be provided, such that the person could be transported upstairs, transferred to a wheelchair at the top of the stairs, and then be either taken or take themselves to the bathroom. Clearly, these three options would involve different activities by different people at different levels. The ultimate aim would be the same, but the impact on the disabled person and family would be quite different.

Handicap is quite the most difficult domain to address, as it varies from person to person, according to their circumstances, and is often outside the control of the health-based rehabilitation team. In terms of the disabled person's life satisfaction, it is the most important area and is the most difficult to measure. Handicap is not an inevitable and direct consequence of impairment and disability. It actually arises from an interaction of the impairment and the disability with other external factors, such as the home environment, the job, personal relations, etc. Its impact derives from society's general attitude to disabled people and it is influenced by culture and by society's values and expectations. For instance, the expectations of the parents of disabled adolescents are significantly lower where there is a congenital disability (or one from a very early age) compared to an acquired disability. The impact of a physical disability on the life of an individual is therefore not just related to the disease process or to the number of individual disabilities, but to what are termed handicap dimensions. These include orientation, physical independence, mobility, occupation, social integration, and economic self-sufficiency and Badley's model (1995) capsulates this (Fig. 2 1). Many people can be severely affected by disability, but are quite satisfied with their lifestyles, whereas others, with similar or lesser disabilities, may be unable to exist

Because handicap is difficult to measure, it is useful to single out these individual dimensions, so that their various elements can be studied further.

Orientation

The impact of a loss of orientation will be seen not only in a decrease in physical independence but in a decrease in social integration and occupation. Orientation involves an awareness of time, place, person, and situation, and when it

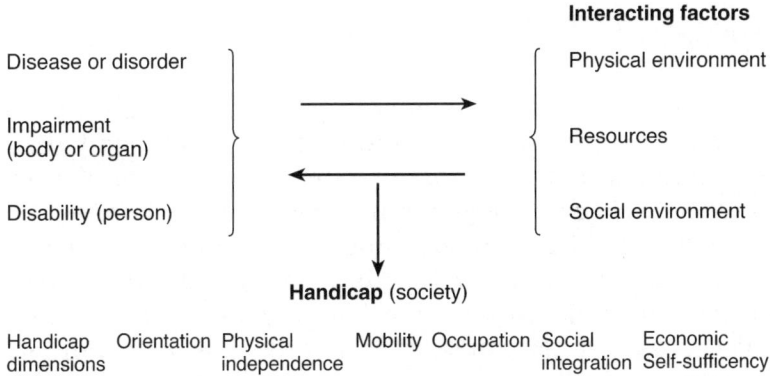

Figure 2.1 A model for the consequences of disease, disorders, or injuries (after Badley and Tennant 1997).

starts to fail, difficulties with the last are often the most obvious. However, it is difficult to measure at a handicap level and qualitative images are often the most appropriate here. For instance, the general tidiness and grooming of a person compared with images from old photographs can be quite revealing. Even in people with newly acquired disabilities, such as someone with a severe traumatic brain injury, reference to photographs is often a good indicator of their persona and their new situation.

Physical independence

This element describes the ability of the individual to make choices. While it is relatively easy to measure independence in terms of personal and domestic activities of daily living, it is recognized that we all need help to live in society. The opportunities that are taken are the essential measures of physical independence, which may be more relevant and perhaps relate to the locus of personal control. However, they are again hard to measure and rehabilitationists find it easier to focus on areas where practical help may be needed. Going through a daily routine of activities is a useful way to identify health needs and the areas where personal and domestic help is required.

....

Mobility

The mobility element in handicap reflects the ability for disabled people to move around their homes and their communities. This therefore may be related to ambulation, to wheelchair use, the geography, and social environment, or to the use of private and public transport. All have an equally important role in assisting mobility. While for some people, the ability to get around may be restricted by purely physical factors, for others, their mobility may be disturbed, for instance, by the fact that their neighbourhood is just not safe. However, for physically disabled people, the ability to get out, either with or without help, can be fairly well measured and this has been done by the OPCS and by its Canadian equivalent survey (HALS). About 22 per cent of disabled adults in the UK survey were restricted to their homes without help and this included 8 per cent of all disabled adults who were considered housebound, even when help was at hand.

Occupation

The occupation activities need not necessarily solely concern paid employment to be consistent with the individual's age, sex, and culture and includes recreation, domestic tasks, vocational and voluntary work, as well as paid employment. Sadly, for many people, paid employment is not an option, not so much because of their disability, but because many live in areas of relatively high unemployment and are subject to the vagaries of prejudices and working practices.

Occupational studies have shown that attending a rehabilitation centre with a specific interest in vocational rehabilitation tends to achieve better results in finding work than in other situations. Similarly, the OPCS survey showed that only 11 per cent of disabled adults (virtually all female) were engaged in home-making. One in 100 were in full-time education and 1 in 3 reported that they were primarily unable to work. The difficulty with many studies is that they do not focus on the younger disabled adult and figures are thus not related to those who would actually be eligible for paid employment.

Social integration

The capacity for social integration depends on a combination of physical independence, mobility, and financial ability. Many people with disabilities live alone and thus social isolation becomes a considerable problem. The OPCS survey reported that 15 per cent of disabled people receive visitors only once a month and 15 per cent reported that they themselves went out less than once a week. The ability to mix socially is also dependent on culture and sex, although there will hopefully be a noticeable change in the opportunities available to women.

Economic self-sufficiency

This is defined as an individual's ability to sustain customary socioeconomic activity and independence. Among people of working age, the OPCS survey found that 72 per cent had income levels less than that of the general population and the proportion of their income gained from employment decreased as the severity of disability increased. As a result, many people are dependent on benefits and have to utilize their income to meet the extra expenses incurred by their disability. The survey found that the largest proportion of the income of poorest families were related to expenditure due to the disability and they were further disadvantaged by this in the wake of other economic pointers.

There is much to be done in the field of independent living for disabled people and knowledge of the factors that disadvantage them is vital. The Disability Discrimination Act 1996 has made a start in identifying areas where improvement is required in our society's approach to disability. Disability is a feature in all our lives (whether personal or through contact) and that health, social, and vocational rehabilitation can make a significant difference to the role of disabled people in our communities. Interventions at the impairment and disability level fall within medical rehabilitation, but these must go hand in hand with reducing the burden of handicap experienced by disabled people. Only that way can expectations rise among disabled people, to allow them to play a full part in society.

Conclusions

Disability is common. About 14 per cent of the adult population of the UK has a disability. Most disability is due to musculo-skeletal disease but neurological problems, whilst giving rise to less disability overall, generally account for the more severely disabling conditions, particularly in younger people. However, disability is common as age increases and older people are more likely to have more than one disabling condition. The prevalence of different disabilities can vary from locality to locality and the prevalence of handicap will alter according to the local services and support networks. Thus, a rehabilitation service should be based on good quality local statistics.

Further reading

Bone, M. and Meltzer, H. (1989). *The prevalence of disability among children*, OPCS Report 3. HMSO, London.

Martin, J., Meltzer, H., and Elliot D. (1988). *The prevalence of disability among adults*, OPCS Report 1. HMSO, London.

3

The rehabilitation team

Multidisciplinary versus interdisciplinary

Rehabilitation is about teamwork. It is a process that has to involve a wide range of professionals. Many teams will be hospital based and working in the post-acute setting and mainly involve physicians, therapists, and nurses. However, other disability teams can work within different contexts and team membership may have a different emphasis. A community rehabilitation team is more likely to involve local authority employees, particularly social workers and community occupational therapists and perhaps other professionals, such as employment experts. Thus, it is not possible or desirable to define disciplines that must be members of a rehabilitation team. This chapter will not produce a tedious list of different disciplines and outline their role. The role of the different professionals should be clear from the context of other chapters in this book. A list of disciplines will inappropriately emphasize professional boundaries. The goal setting process needs to be clearly focused towards the disabled person and their own aims and aspirations. Sometimes these goals will cross discipline boundaries and will need to be enacted through a number of different professionals working together towards the same end. For example, a short-term goal may be for the person to negotiate a flight of stairs in a particular fashion. It is not just the job of the physiotherapist to assist in this goal. The physiotherapist will advise about the best way to achieve that aim but the implementation is the responsibility of all team members. The speech therapist leading the person to a speech session up a flight of stairs will need to be aware of the stair-climbing technique just as much as the physiotherapist will need to be aware of the communication strategy that is being directed by the speech therapist. Rehabilitation team members will need to be flexible and be prepared to work across artificial professional boundaries. This is the essence of interdisciplinary working. 'That's not my job' is not an attitude required in a rehabilitation team. Thus, interdisciplinary working implies a degree of blurring of professional roles whilst still preserving the separate identity and expertise of individual professions. Multidisciplinary is a term that simply describes a number of different disciplines working with the same disabled person. Rehabilitation is all about interdisciplinary working and not about multidisciplinary working.

Generic rehabilitation therapist?

A logical extension to the interdisciplinary argument is the abandonment of professional disciplines and adoption of the broader concept of a generic rehabilitation therapist. This concept is now being followed by a number of rehabilitation units. For many years physiotherapy, occupational therapy, and other health disciplines have employed assistants who have been through a training course but not at a level to achieve professional status and recognition. These individuals are normally employed to carry out the more routine treatments under the guidance and supervision of a qualified therapist. In some units such individuals now work across professional boundaries and act as generic rehabilitation assistants performing routine tasks under the supervision and guidance of the different professions. There are clear advantages in this system for the disabled person who may be able to develop a better working relationship with a single generic assistant rather than with a range of such assistants and senior professionals. However, at the moment there is no hard evidence that such an approach is better than more traditional approaches.

A logical extension of the generic assistant is a new style degree-trained generic or rehabilitation therapist. The therapist may be guided by other therapy disciplines but would be an autonomous therapist in their own right. Such individuals do not exist in the UK except in a few private units. However, in other countries, such as the United States, and in other contexts, such as the system of conductive education in Hungary, such broader trained professionals do exist. Once again there is no hard evidence at the moment that rehabilitation therapists produce greater benefits but this proposal does have a logic in tune with the philosophy of rehabilitation.

Keyworker or case manager?

Whatever mode of working is adopted by a team there will always be a large number of individuals who will need to liaise with the disabled person. This can produce a sense of confusion or lack of clear direction for the disabled individual. Many teams have got round this problem by adoption of a keyworker system. One team member is allocated to be the key liaison between the team and the disabled person and family. The keyworker will be the main source of information about the rehabilitation process and feed back the thoughts and aspirations of the disabled person to the team and vice versa. This is not a substitute for regular whole team meetings nor should there be an abrogation of responsibility by relevant professionals. It is simply a system that leads to better coordination and liaison and which should ensure clear communication.

The role of the keyworker can be extended to that of the case manager. The role of the case manager is outlined in more detail in Chapter 4.

Core team and network team

Despite the importance of interdisciplinary working and the necessity of breaking down artificial professional boundaries there is a core membership for a health-orientated rehabilitation team. Core members of the team would include:
- rehabilitation physician
- rehabilitation nurses
- clinical neuropsychologist
- occupational therapist
- physiotherapist
- speech and language therapist.

It would be difficult to envisage a rehabilitation team that does not have access to such individuals. The team would clearly need to draw on a wide range of other expertise, particularly a social worker and a counsellor, and part-time access to a dietician, chiropodist, and rehabilitation engineer. Access to other medical specialities, particularly urology and orthopaedic surgery, would be essential. A broader team, or at least a broader network of individuals, is required for a rehabilitation team with a community focus. Health requirements quickly change into social requirements and input from social service occupational therapists and social workers is soon needed. Useful links can be fostered with employment rehabilitation experts and, according to local availability, to other voluntary providers, lawyers, the local social security office, and a variety of disability support groups. The success of a team is often dependent on the network of personal contacts rather than actual team membership.

What constitutes a team?

A team is more than a collection of individuals conveniently grouped together into a working relationship. Characteristics of a team have been defined by Furnell:[1]
- professionals from different disciplines meeting regularly

- agreement on explicit objectives for the team which determine the team structure and function
- the allocation of a significant proportion of time to the pursuit of these objectives
- adequate administrative and clinical coordination to support the work of the team
- a defined geographical base
- a clear differentiation of and respect for those skills and roles which are specifically unique to individual members as well as recognition of those roles which may be shared.

Key factors are having a team identity, spending time on development of the team, sharing goals and objectives for the team, and having a place to meet and discuss such issues. The team needs to determine its fundamental philosophical stance and to agree clear admission criteria, modes of referral, details of process, outcome measures, and discharge criteria. Such basic 'rules' are important to maintain a clear team identity for both internal and external perception.

Time for team building is important and most established teams now recommend that the team as a whole has a day off at least once a year in a separate environment to review progress and for mutual encouragement, praise, and criticism. The maintenance of team cohesion by such team building is just as important as the creation of the team in the first place.

Team leadership

This can be problematic. Leadership of many rehabilitation teams is by the doctor. This is usually for historical or political reasons and not necessarily because the doctor makes the best leader. Indeed it can be argued that the medical training by its very nature encourages autonomous independent thinking in order to make quick decisions in acute situations and that this style is not best suited to the qualities required from a team leader. Within some organizations it is still not practical to suggest that anyone other than the doctor should lead the team. Physicians do have advantages as medicine is one of the few specialities able to give a broad overview of a particular disorder rather than the narrower perspective of other professional disciplines. This ability to have a view of the 'whole person' with some grasp of the role of the other professionals can be a helpful leadership characteristic. However, ideally the team leader should have the necessary characteristics of a leader. There is much literature on this subject. A leader has been described as 'someone tolerant enough to listen to others but strong enough to reject their advice'.[2] A leader will clearly need interpersonal and social skills, have some vision for the long-term future of the team, and the ability to communicate that vision yet remain flexible enough to adjust the direction according to the thoughts and views of other team members. The leader should be tough enough to make difficult decisions as and when they arise. Organizational skills are required as well as enough time to devote to team activities. Finally, in the modern NHS it is useful for the team leader to have a grasp of finance and budgetary control as well as the necessary political skills to influence colleagues and managers and direct maximum resources to the team. It is doubtful whether an individual exists who can fulfil all these criteria!

Conclusions

Rehabilitation is team work. Although the team will consist of a number of core disciplines, it must work in a interdisciplinary manner and be prepared to cross professional boundaries. The team will need to involve a broad network of other individuals in order to give maximum benefit to the disabled person. It will need time to devote to team activities and team building and will need to have a clearly defined and agreed set of goals and objectives as well as a system that is robust enough to monitor performance and a willingness to adjust goals and objectives according to that performance. Every team needs a leader, who may be the rehabilitation physician, but who must have the necessary leadership skills, including vision, respect of and for other team members, flexibility, and determination. The right team with the right leader is the key to rehabilitation.

References

1. Furnell, J., Flett, S., and Clarke, D. F. (1987). Multidisciplinary clinical teams: some issues in establishment and function. *Hospital & Health Services Review*, January, 15–18.
2. Belbin, R. M. (1981). *Management teams*. Heinemann, London.

Further reading

Brill, N. I. (1976). *Team work: working together in human services*. Lipincott, Philadelphia.
Dyer, W. G. (1984). *Team building: issues and alternatives*. Addison-Wesley, Reading, MA.
Vroom, V. H., and Yetton, P. W. (1973). *Leadership and decision making*. University of Pittsburgh Press, Pittsburgh.
Wood, R. (1993). The rehabilitation team. In: Greenwood, R., Barnes, M. P., McMillan, T. M., and Ward, C. D. (ed.) *Neurological rehabilitation*, pp.41–9. Churchill Livingstone, London.

4

....

Organization of services

This chapter will discuss various organizational aspects of the delivery of a rehabilitation service. The previous chapter has discussed the composition of the rehabilitation team and the team dynamics as well as questions of leadership. The rehabilitation team must, however, work within a structural context. It must liaise effectively with local and regional colleagues within the health service as well as a variety of other professionals in the statutory, voluntary, and private sectors. In addition there are a number of philosophical approaches to the structural organization of disability services which will need to be addressed. Overall, this chapter will outline some of the options available and discuss the merits and drawbacks of some of these possibilities. The local situation will vary from country to country and it is not possible in this chapter to provide a comprehensive review of service organization around the world. The chapter, of necessity, will tend to concentrate on services in the United Kingdom and regrettably needs to have an emphasis on services within the developed world.

Principles of service delivery

The first step for a team is to agree on the basic principles on which the work is to be based. There are many different foundations varying from principles based on the medical model of disability on the one hand to the social model of disability on the other. A set of principles that is now gaining broad acceptance are those devised by the Prince of Wales Advisory Group on Disability in 1985. These principles can be summarized as follows:

1. Consultation with disabled people and their families on services as they are planned.
2. Information clearly presented and readily available to all disabled consumers.
3. Articipation of disabled people in the life of local and national committees with respect to both responsibilities and benefits.
4. Choice as to where to live and how to maintain independence including help in learning how to choose.
5. Recognition that long-term disability is not synonymous with illness and that the medical model of care is inappropriate in the majority of cases.
6. Autonomy for the freedom to make decisions regarding a way of life best suited to an individual disabled person's circumstances.

An agreement on such principles upon which the team will operate will help to determine the structure in which the team wishes to work and also help to define the nature of the liaison and cooperation with other health professionals and disabled people.

Specific service requirements

There is now, across much of the developed world, a general agreement that there should be a two-tier rehabilitation service. Most rehabilitation can and should be carried out either at home or in the individual's own locality. Thus, a fundamental prerequisite is for the presence of an accessible local rehabilitation team. However, it is also recognized that a minority of disabled people, probably around 10 per cent, will require the expertise and facilities of a more specialist service. Thus, at least throughout Europe, we are seeing the beginnings of a network of regional specialist rehabilitation centres which are developing close links with a broader network of local rehabilitation and disability teams. The range of services required at a regional level and local level will clearly depend on availability of staff, resources, and facilities and will obviously vary from area to area. However, there is some consensus on the general scope of services that are likely to be needed within a specialist rehabilitation centre and at a local level.

Regional specialist rehabilitation centres

There is a need for specialist centres serving a population of about three million people. Such centres should run along the same interdisciplinary lines as the local rehabilitation unit and will need to maintain very close links with the local network. Ideally, specialist centres should be seen as a resource to be used by disabled people, their keyworkers, and therapists to learn from the expertise contained within the centre and to make use of specialist equipment and facilities. The centre should act as a focus for education, training, and research both for local rehabilitation teams and other colleagues. Specific services that should be provided from a specialist centre should include:

- A specialist rehabilitation service for the people with the most complex, often multiple, disabilities, particularly including those with brain damage who have a combination of physical, psychological, and behavioural problems.
- A specialist service for complex wheelchair and special seating requirements.
- A bioengineering service.
- A communication aids centre.
- An information, advice, and assessment service for car driving.
- An amputee service.
- A spinal injury service—the UK has seen the development of a network of separate spinal injury centres but there is no reason why such centres should not be incorporated within a broader specialist rehabilitation service and thus able to draw on a wide range of specialist expertise.

Finally, there is a need to consider regional provision of residential care for the most severely disabled people who cannot realistically be looked after in the community. This population is likely to include those in persistent vegetative state or in prolonged coma. There are very few such people but nevertheless their quality of life does depend on a very high standard of specialist nursing and therapy.

Local specialist rehabilitation service

The local rehabilitation team should be able to deliver post-acute in-patient rehabilitation for individuals after, for example, stroke or head injury, as well as being able to deliver community support for those with residual disabilities or ongoing progressive conditions, such as multiple sclerosis. It is likely that such a team will need to have a hospital base with in-patient facilities but should be able to work within the local community as well. Unfortunately, in the UK, the recent changes in the National Health Service have forced a rather artificial split between acute Trusts and community-based Trusts and has made this seamless delivery of rehabilitation services much more difficult to achieve. However, it is hoped that the new changes proposed for the National Health Service in terms of better cooperation and partnership between purchasers and providers of health care will lead to smoother delivery of services across hospital and community boundaries.

In specific terms the local rehabilitation team should be able to provide a basic rehabilitation service including a continence service, an orthotic service, a pressure sore service, a prescription and maintenance service for basic wheelchairs, and a counselling service, particularly sexual counselling. It is likely that these services will fall within the remit of health authority or primary care group of purchase. Other services that will need to be provided at a local level should be purchased and provided on a joint basis between health authority and local authorities. Such services could include an aids and equipment display and loan facility, perhaps contained within a disabled living centre, an information service and access to a broad range of housing, respite, and day-centre facilities. Ideally a comprehensive rehabilitation team should include members who are employed by social services such as community occupational therapists and social workers.

Rehabilitation unit

It would be possible for a rehabilitation team to be based either within the community or even within a hospital but without direct access to beds. The team could simply offer support and advice to disabled people directly on medical or surgical wards. However, there are clear advantages to the creation of a dedicated rehabilitation unit. The physical structure of the unit could be made more conducive to rehabilitation by the provision of, for example, a broader range of communal living spaces, practice kitchen, bedroom, and living areas and even self-contained flats to allow further practice of daily living skills. The team approach is likely to be facilitated within a physical unit, the staff morale should be higher, research can be stimulated, and voluntary help is more likely. The geographical site of the unit is probably less important than the internal design. However, there are probably psychological advantages in moving from an acute hospital site to a separate rehabilitation site as a step towards a return to the community. Obviously units should be accessible to public transport and within or close to a local community setting in order to allow functional goals to be introduced in a realistic community environment. The number of beds required in a unit will clearly vary according to population served, admission and discharge policy, and diagnostic criteria. As a very broad estimate around 20 beds would normally be required to meet the post-acute rehabilitation needs of the 16–65-year-old population with neurological disabilities within a population of around 250 000 people. However, it is still important to emphasize that much of the work of a local rehabilitation team can and should be carried out within the community. Logistics and time may dictate that some therapy sessions will need to be carried out in a group setting but again this need not be within a hospital but can be more appropriately provided within, for example, a general practitioner's surgery, a community centre, church hall, or leisure complex.

Models of service delivery

Chapter 2 has demonstrated that about 14 per cent of the adult population have a disability and at least 2–3 per cent of the population have a severe disability. The adequate and equitable delivery of health care to the disabled population is clearly a major logistical problem. There is also no doubt that at the present time the service provided in most countries is patchy, fragmented, and overall inadequate. What service delivery options are available?

Medical clinics

The traditional model is for the longer-term management of people with disabilities to be through the hospital out-patient clinic. This is unsatisfactory. There is often little continuity of care with follow-up visits supervised by junior medical staff with little knowledge of the individual and indeed often with little knowledge of disability. The numbers of people involved means that little time can be spent with any one person and the re-appointment intervals will tend to be long. This model provides little or no involvement by members of a rehabilitation team. It may have some relevance in certain conditions such as epilepsy or Parkinson's disease, but in general fails to meet the principles of service delivery outlined above and is widely known to be an unsatisfactory experience both for the doctor and disabled person.

Disease-specific clinics

There is a recent trend towards establishment of disease-specific clinics such as for multiple sclerosis, epilepsy, or Parkinson's disease. These clinics certainly have the advantage of providing an expert multidisciplinary team familiar with the specific problems of that disorder. The team can supply information and counselling support and can act as a focus for self-help groups. Thus, the clinic could provide a social as well as medical function. In addition research can be facilitated. However, there are logistical problems of arranging a large number of such clinics to cover the whole range of disabilities and the distinct possibility of ignoring the needs of disabled people with rarer conditions. There is also the real danger of staff boredom and the problem of individuals seeing others with the same condition who are worse than themselves with the consequent psychological stress both for them and their carers.

Community rehabilitation teams

It is obviously possible for the acute rehabilitation and hospital-based team to remain in touch with the disabled person after discharge. This will provide continuity of support and access to appropriate health resources. However, a single disability team in a district would soon be overwhelmed by the numbers of people that need to be seen. Regular review for large numbers of people would quickly place an unacceptable demand on the service. Some centres operate an open access service for self re-referral which can counteract this problem. However, a self-referral review system can mean that preventable complications arise unrecognized by the disabled person. Such a post-acute rehabilitation team continuing an overview can also have the disadvantage of having a health orientation with the potential to ignore important social and vocational aspects of disability. There are examples of broader-based multidisciplinary teams with input from social services, employment, and other voluntary and statutory bodies. This requires a great deal of coordination and cooperation between different statutory and funding agencies and, at least within the present UK system, is difficult to achieve.

Primary care team

A typical group general practice in the UK has a population of around 10 000. The numbers of disabled people are thus reduced within a primary care practice to a reasonable level. It is possible for the primary care team to keep a watching brief on the disabled people and make referrals to a local hospital-based team as appropriate. However, many disabilities are quite rare. For example, a general practitioner is likely to see only one new person with multiple sclerosis every 20 years. The level of expertise within the primary care team is limited and important points of management may be missed and questions left unanswered. It is likely that a system dependent on a primary care team will produce a rather uncoordinated and fragmented service. In order to get around this problem there are some examples of the primary care team being supported by visiting members of a specialist rehabilitation team. In one project a rehabilitation consultant and physiotherapist attended meetings of the primary care team to discuss management issues for people with Parkinson's disease. Such projects have potential but need further evaluation.

Case manager

Disabled people, particularly those with severe and wide ranging disabilities, will need a complex array of health and social services. The concept of case management has been developed as a way of assisting disabled people with the coordination of the necessary professional staff. Case management can include:

- simple coordination within a single agency
- coordination across agency boundaries
- service brokerage in which the case manager negotiates with the key agencies on the client's behalf
- budget holding responsibility where services can be purchased on behalf of the client from statutory bodies or other voluntary or private agencies.

There have been very few controlled studies of the efficacy of case management but it is widely practised within the USA and Canada and probably provides a better and more coherent service, particularly for those who have a degree of cognitive impairment who are unable to find their own way through the maze of services.

Nurse practitioner

Recently the concept of the specialist nurse has evolved. Often such nurses are hospital based and have developed expertise in particular conditions such as Parkinson's disease, epilepsy, and multiple sclerosis. Some studies have demonstrated clear benefit from a specialist nurse both working in the community and from hospital. One study evaluating a multiple sclerosis liaison nurse in the community demonstrated a higher rate of appropriate referral to other therapists and improved coping, mood, confidence, and knowledge of multiple sclerosis among the client group. Carers also reported similar subjective benefits and general practitioners found the scheme to be helpful. Much of the benefit probably derives from the keyworker or case manager role but it can be a method of introducing community-based care with expertise and back-up from appropriate medical or other staff. Often such individuals are trained in counselling skills which is a much undervalued role in community services.

Independent Living Movement

A logical extension of a case manager is the disabled person or family themselves carrying out this role. There are now examples of local authorities giving disabled people their own budget to buy in services as required. This is a model that is firmly supported by the Independent Living Movement and by disabled groups in general. It is certainly a workable and practical solution for certain groups of disabled people, particularly for those who are cognitively intact. It becomes a difficult system when one is dealing with cognitive disturbance. Who should manage the affairs of those who are unable to do so? How does one deal with inappropriate or unprovidable purchasing requests? What happens if the disabled person is not able to handle the budgeting arrangements adequately? What guide-lines and safety nets need to be introduced? This is certainly a model worthy of consideration but is not applicable to, nor wanted by, all disabled people.

Resource centre

A model of delivery that could overcome some of the difficulties outlined in the other models is the creation of community resource centres. Such centres would be local, accessible, and could house a range of facilities including an information service, disabled living centre, act as a base for self-help groups, and as a physical site for the local rehabilitation team. It would be possible for out-patient clinics from the local hospital to be held within such a centre and for social and recreational activities to be organized in or from the centre. Other agencies could be involved such as housing, social security, and employment. The centres could be managed by disabled people with the support of appropriate health and local authority personnel. Some centres have now been established along these lines in the UK and seem to offer a potential solution to the problems of service delivery. In particular such centres help to form close partnerships between disabled people and health and social professionals.

Community-based rehabilitation in developing countries

Most of the above models are not applicable in the developing world. Rehabilitation resources in many developing countries are non-existent or only exist in regional, often private, centres. Developing countries have very few trained therapists, nurses, or doctors working within the rehabilitation field. Those that are employed often remain within the larger urban centres of population leaving vast numbers of disabled people in rural communities without access to any services at all. In response to this problem the World Health Organization has developed the concept of community-based rehabilitation (CBR). The CBR model is open to a number of different interpretations. The most accepted model is that the local community should be the main supporters of their own disabled population (Fig. 4.1). Local village workers, often those involved in child birth and basic health care, can be given further disability training. There are a number of training courses around the world often supported and sponsored by non-governmental organizations. It has been demonstrated that a reasonable training in disability, given to someone with background health knowledge, can be delivered in around 6–8 weeks. Individuals with this period of training can, albeit at a very basic level, cope with the needs of around 80 per cent of the disabled population. Obviously the village workers will need intermittent support and ongoing training from a central organization. Access will be required, if at all possible, to regional urban centres. The disabled people in a given village or locality are encouraged to form self-help groups for information sharing, peer support, and for employment. There are many examples of disabled village groups who have banded together to provide an economically viable employment such as wood working and dress making. Many groups contribute a small sum to a central pool so that the few members of the group needing medicines or referral can afford such intervention. In other models 'camps' are organized in villages where the local disability team provides a regular 'out-patient' session. Unfortunately there is very little research into appropriate models in the developing world and no clear consensus on appropriate training programmes and ongoing support. Much more needs to be done on a global basis and significant investment is required in developing countries into an appropriate disability and rehabilitation infrastructure.

Liaison

It is clear from this book that longer-term rehabilitation support goes well beyond the boundaries of health care. Many different departments in the local authority such as housing and social services have an important role to play as does social security, employment, and a variety of other voluntary and private agencies. The problems of disability in the longer term are generally those of coordination between these different bodies. There is an overwhelming need for close and formal liaison between the different individuals involved. Preferably we should be working towards provision of services purchased jointly by the relevant statutory bodies and provided by a single coherent

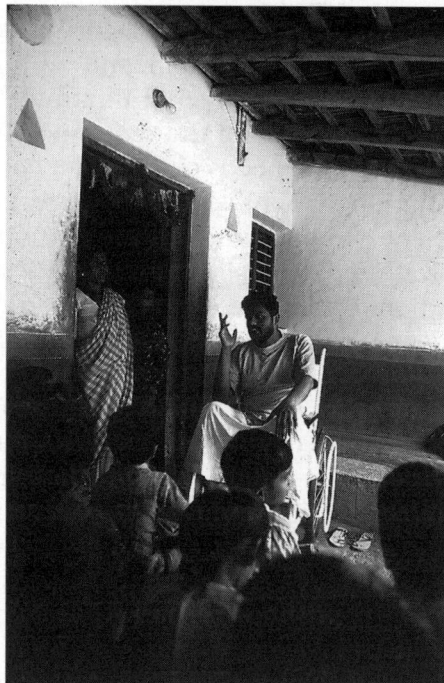

Fig. 4.1 A disabled person working in the local community in rural India.

organization. Fortunately in the UK the government has recently proposed easing the legislation around funding for health and social services which should make joint working more achievable in the near future. It is also important to emphasize that organizations of disabled people and disabled people themselves must be involved in the planning, management, and in the delivery of rehabilitation and disability services.

Conclusions

There is no single prescriptive model for the organization of disability services. The model depends on local facilities, resources, potential team membership, and the degree of cooperation and liaison between the different statutory bodies including health services, social services, and the education and employment sector. However, there is now a consensus that there should be a two-tier rehabilitation system—a regional specialist centre serving the needs of people with complex or rarer conditions while complementing the local rehabilitation services who should deal with the majority of the day-to-day problems of disabled people. Both regional and local services would benefit from in-patient facilities but the local team undoubtedly needs a strong community focus. A number of different models of service are outlined but throughout the benefit of close liaison with a wide network of professional agencies and with the disabled people themselves must be emphasized. Rehabilitation will only work if it is a real partnership between professionals and their disabled clientele.

Further reading

British Society of Rehabilitation Medicine (1992). *Neurological rehabilitation in the United Kingdom—report of a working party.* British Society of Rehabilitation Medicine, London.

British Society of Rehabilitation Medicine (1993). *Advice to purchasers—setting NHS contracts for rehabilitation medicine.* British Society of Rehabilitation Medicine, London.

European Federation of Neurological Societies (1997). Minimum standards for a neurological rehabilitation service. *European Journal of Neurology,* 4, S1–S7.

Helander, E., Mendis, P., Nelson, G., and Goerdt, A. (1989). *Training in the community for people with disabilities.* WHO, Geneva.

Neurological Alliance (1996). *Living with a neurological condition—standards of care.* Neurological Alliance, London.

Neurological Alliance (1996). *Providing a service for people with neurological conditions.* Neurological Alliance, London.

Prince of Wales Advisory Group on Disability (1985). *Living options.* Prince of Wales Advisory Group on Disability, London.

Werner, D. (1988). *Disabled village children.* The Hesperian Foundation, PO Box 1692, Palo Alto, CA 94302, USA.

5

Assessment of disability

Introduction

Rehabilitation is a very complex activity and measurement of outcome lacks the specificity seen in the treatment of pathology. For instance, reducing inflammatory markers in polymyalgia treatment shows that treatment is effective. Many patients following an acute single injury or illness will make a spontaneous recovery or improvement independent of the treatment that is applied. Other patients may have disorders that cause a progressive deterioration, but rehabilitation may slow down the deterioration and improve their quality of life. Simple measures will not show this. There are essentially five categories of patients, which are listed below:

1. Patients who will make a spontaneous, full improvement to return to premorbid levels of health.
2. Patients who will improve steadily but may not return to premorbid levels of health and function and will be helped by rehabilitation.
3. Patients who will not improve greatly, but may be helped by rehabilitation.
4. Patients who will deteriorate slowly, but this deterioration will be slowed by treatment and rehabilitation.
5. Patients who will progress steadily or rapidly despite any rehabilitation input.

Rehabilitation can therefore be effective in categories 2, 3, and 4 and patients may present with very different problems. Managers will wish to see the impact of a rehabilitation episode and outcome measures have become important for assessing patient care as well as for allocating funding for services. Separation of rehabilitation issues into those of pathology, impairments, disability, and handicap are thus important in the measurement of outcome. The ICIDH classification is now becoming more positive, with the 'disability' category being changed to 'functional capacity' or 'abilities' and 'handicap' being defined in terms of 'advantages'.

Measurement

Measurement is the use of a standard to quantify an observation. Measurement tools are the techniques used to quantify that observation and the outcome is the result obtained in using such instruments. It is very convenient to enumerate scales, but there are certain aspects of rehabilitation, which are difficult to put into an ordinal or hierarchical fashion. The essential measure in rehabilitation is to define the goals of rehabilitation for a particular patient and to determine whether or not the patient achieved the goal at the end of the rehabilitation episode. This is a measure of success, but the true value depends on the skill of the team in defining realistic, achievable, and desirable targets. If a goal is too easy, then the measure will have a ceiling effect, i.e. too many people will achieve the goal or the top of the scale, whereas if it is too difficult, the patient's actual achievements will not be amply recognized.

Linear quantitative measures are obviously useful and five categories are described—nominal, ordinal, interval, ratio, and hierarchical. *Nominal scales* classify a characteristic number along a straight line. Points on the scale have no meaning within the context in which they are being used, but may be useful if the frequencies of that particular characteristic are being studied. An *ordinal scale* ranks the order, so that each adjacent score measures a parameter along a line, i.e. one point above or below is higher or lower than the last. The visual analogue scale is typical of this and the Barthel Index and Functional Independence Measurements are good examples of ordinal scales. *Interval scales* are truly useful as quantitative scales, in that the interval is common and there is a constant unit of measurement between one point and another on the linear scale. The zero point is quite arbitrary, as perhaps are the units of measurement. A *ratio scale* is an integral scale with a true zero at its origin. Measuring weight for example would describe a ratio scale. Many measures in health economics, such as cost per case, are also of this type. *Hierarchical scales* show a natural hierarchy of assets, such that each point on the rise of a scale indicates a greater ability or skill than the last.

The ideal scale should be sensitive, specific, reliable, appropriate, acceptable, and robust. Each must be validated against standard criteria to which the attribute may be assessed. Many disability measures have not been validated and value of their robustness is required not only as a general measure, but as a measure of specific rehabilitation activity, e.g. the Barthel ADL Index in stroke rehabilitation. In disability research, false positive and false negative findings are common and a true positive rate (the sensitivity) needs to be compared against the false positive rate (i.e. the specificity). Not only must scores be valid, they must also be reliable and consistent and reliable *between* raters as well as repeatable, so inter-rater reliability and test–retest reliability are of importance. They must also be robust enough to be worthy of comment and therefore the simpler they are, the better.

Impairment, disability, and handicap

These terms are defined at the start of the book. Measures have also been organized around these domains and it is worth looking at them further in this context.

Measures of impairment

These are more likely to be reasonably objective and they

are easier to record in simple scales compared to disability and handicap measures.

Mobility
Accurate measures of muscle power can be determined using a dynamometer. However, while this is accurate, information on patients' ability to stand and walk is not particularly useful. The MRC scale is an ordinal scale, but is not sensitive enough to be of much use in neurological or musculoskeletal rehabilitation. One can communicate to other professionals the degree of weakness, but there are large variations in the levels of the scale. This is so much the case that some clinicians have introduced sub-divisions within the level, using plus and minus signs. The MRC scale is described in Table 5.1. The scale can be used in all upper and lower limb muscle groups and is more useful in peripheral neuropathies, where one may wish to measure single features of muscle weakness.

In neurological rehabilitation, spasticity is a major potential complication and can be measured using the Modified Ashworth Scale. Although it is also crude, it is the best clinical tool to date. The Wortenburg's pendular test is more accurate, but is clinically less practical. For ambulant children with cerebral palsy, the state of the child's maturation is an added complication for which the Rosenbaum developmental scale probably produces the

Table 5.1 MRC scale

0	No muscular activity
1	Minimal contraction of muscle but insufficient to move a joint
2	Contraction of muscle sufficient to move a joint but not oppose gravity
3	Muscle contraction sufficient to move a joint against gravity, but not against physical resistance
4	Muscle contraction sufficient to move a joint against gravity and against mild/moderate resistance
5	Normal power, i.e. muscular contraction sufficient to resist firm resistance

best assessment battery. Table 5.2 describes the Modified Ashworth Scale.

Where walking is possible, one of the simplest and most accurate measures is to measure the speed of walking over a set distance or a set time. Both are valid and reliable. In addition, a 'time to get up and go' test, which includes the time taken to rise from a chair and start walking as well as the speed of walking is also a valid assessment. The Motricity Index is a useful measure of limb impairment and divides into a lower limb section and an upper limb section. It is now widely used in clinical practice to record recovery after stroke and is described in Table 5.3.

Upper limb and hand function
The arm's prehensile function can be assessed in many ways. Dynamometer grip strength is fairly crude, but is simple to perform. However, grip strength using a small cuff and sphygmomanometer is useful in clinical practice. The nine-hole peg test reflects the ability to perform coordinated fine movements rather than grasp. The patient is asked to place nine wooden pegs, each 9 mm in diameter and 32 mm long into a corresponding number of holes, which are spaced 15 mm apart in three rows of three. The time taken to place the pegs in the holes is recorded, but the test should be terminated if it is not completed in 50 seconds. Recording the number of pegs placed at this

Table 5.2 Modified Ashworth scale. Adapted from Bohannon and Smith.[1]

4	Rigid extremity
3	Loss of full joint movement, difficult movement, considerable tone
2	Full joint/limb movement, but more marked increase in tone, limb still easily moved
1+	Slight increase in tone, catch and resistance throughout range of movement
1	Slight increase in tone, catch, or minimal resistance at end of range of movement
0	No increase in tone

....

Table 5.3   Motricity index

		Tests (in a sitting position)
Arm	1	Pinchgrip : 2.5cm cube between thumb and forefinger
	2	Elbow flexion, from 90°, voluntary contraction/ movement
	3	Shoulder abduction : from against chest
Leg	4	Ankle dorsiflexion : from plantar flexed position
	5	Knee extension : from 90°, voluntary contraction/ movement
	6	Hip flexion : usually from 90°

Scoring
Test 1 (Pinchgrip)
 0: No movement
11: Beginnings of prehension (any movement of finger or thumb)
19: Grips cube, but unable to hold against gravity
22: Grips cube, held against gravity but not against weak pull
26: Grips cube against pull, but weaker than other side
33: Normal pinchgrip

Tests 2 to 6
 0: No movement
 9: Palpable contraction in muscle but no movement
14: Movement seen but not full range/not against gravity
19: Movement : full range against gravity, not against resistance.
25: Movement against resistance, but weaker than other side
33: Normal power

Arm score = scores (1) + (2) + (3) + 1 (to make 100)
Leg score = scores (4) + (5) + (6) + 1 (to make 100)
Side score = (arm plus leg) 2

Guidelines
The patient should be sitting in a chair or on the edge of a bed, but can be
tested lying if necessary. The grading is derived from the Medical
Research Council (MRC) grades but weighted scores are used. Six limbs
are tested.

Pinchgrip
Ask the patient to grip a 2.5 cm object (cubed) between thumb and
forefinger. Objects should be on a flat surface. Monitor any forearm or
small hand muscle.
19 = Drops object when lifted (examiner may need to lift wrist).
22 = Can hold in air but easily dislodged.

Elbow flexion
Elbow flexed to 90°, forearm horizontal and upper arm vertical. Patient
asked to bend elbows so that hand touches shoulder. Examiner resists
with hand on wrist. Monitor biceps.
14 = If no movement seen, may hold elbow out so that arm is horizontal.

Shoulder abduction with elbow fully flexed and against chest
Patient asked to abduct arm. Monitor contraction of deltoid; movement of shoulder girdle does not count—there must be movement of humerus in relation to scapula.
19 = Adducted more than 90°, beyond horizontal.

Ankle dorsiflexion
Foot relaxed in plantar flexed position. Patient asked to dorsiflex foot. Monitor tibialis anterior.
14 = Less than full range of dorsiflexion.

Knee extension
Foot unsupported, knee at 90°. Patient asked to extend knee to touch examiner's hand held level with the knee. Monitor contraction of quadriceps.
14 = Less than 50% of full extension (i.e. 45°).
19 = Knee fully extended but easily pushed down.

Hip flexion
Sitting with hip bent at 90°. Patient asked to lift knee towards chin. Check for associated movement of leaning back by placing hand behind back and asking patient not to lean back. Monitor contraction of ileopsoas.
14 = Less than full range of possible flexion (check passive movement).
19 = Fully flexed but easily pushed down

time is also valid. It is useful in both neurological and musculoskeletal rehabilitation. In addition, the arm section of the Motricity Index is widely used in clinical practice.

Functional activity
Many people with disabilities can actually carry out tasks, but are greatly fatigued by them. The effort required to carry out daily living activities is difficult to measure, but the nearest approximation comes from measuring the heart rate, which is used in the calculation of a physiological cost index (PCI). Oxygen consumption can be measured using breathing masks and Douglas bags, or more specialized equipment in a laboratory, but this is of little use in clinical situations. PCI is useful for both ambulant people and for wheelchair users and I s calculated in the following way:

$$PCI = \frac{\text{Pulse rate during activity } - \text{ pulse rate}}{\text{Speed of activity}}$$

Communication

Dysphasia can be screened using the Frenchay Asphasia Screening Test (FAST). This is the ability to record a set of pictures and is clinically a useful bedside test. It correlates with the Boston Aphasia Screening Test, which is regularly used by speech and language therapists.

Cognitive measures

The Mini-Mental State Examination is widely used as screening test of cognitive impairment. It includes an assessment of many elements of higher cerebral functions, such as memory, attention, and language. It is a useful basic tool for inclusion in a battery of tests of cognitive function. However, the Hodkinson Mental Test and the digit span, which is a test of attention within the Weschler Adult Intelligence Scale (WAIS), are valuable at the bedside. With the Hodkinson score the patient scores 1 for correct answers to the following questions:

• Age of patient
• Time (to nearest hour)
• An address given for recall at end of test
• Name of hospital (or area of town if patient is at home)
• Year
• Patient's date of birth
• Month
• Dates of significant event, e.g. Second World War
• Name of Monarch/Prime Minister
• Count backwards from 20 to 1 (no errors but may correct self).

The Hospital Anxiety and Depression Scale is relevant in physical disability, since there is little chance of inappropriate responses. It is useful in stroke rehabilitation, but its value diminishes thereafter. A score of 7 or below for anxiety/depression is normal, though scores of 11 or above are abnormal. Similarly, the General Health Questionnaire (GHQ) is widely used and well validated. It is reliable, simple, and easy to apply.

Disability measures

Many measures span impairments and disabilities and the

OPCS Disability Scale is perhaps one of these. It is increasingly widely used. It measures a broad range of mobility activities in both upper and lower limbs. The ability to reach, to stretch and the dexterity sections complement functions associated with ambulation. However, its usage in areas other than rehabilitation units is likely to be small for the time being.

Activities of daily living (ADL)
Of the numerous ADL measures, the best is undoubtedly the Barthel Index and its many modifications. One most commonly used is given in table 5.4. The index is validated in stroke and is predictive at one month for functional independence at six months. It includes ten core areas of activities of daily living. In neurological rehabilitation, its use is hampered by the fact that it does not take into account difficulties with communication, cognition, and mood. Having said that, it is simple, reliable, and quick to carry out. The scale should measure what the patient does do rather than what he or she can do and thus an element of hierarchical significance appears.

The development of neurological rehabilitation has exposed limitations of the Barthel Index and the Functional Independence Measure has thus been developed by Carl Grainger and others. This is now the most widely used measure in rehabilitation units in the United States and is geared towards measuring the burden of care required to maintain a disabled person. There are 18 subsets, which are measured on a scale of 1 to 7 (1 being total care required, to 7 being full independence). Because of the limitations of genuine measures of disability and burden of care in traumatic brain injury, the Functional Assessment Measure (FAM) has been added to the FIM. This uses the same criteria but the FAM measures extend activities of daily living to cover community mobility and cognitive features which are relevant to post-acute traumatic brain injury rehabilitation. The FIM+FAM is only validated for in-patient settings and is designed to be performed by the whole rehabilitation team. It is also designed to give information for the planning of rehabilitation goals and scores can be displayed, in such a way that deficits can be

Table 5.4 The Barthel Index Score (total score up to 20).

Task	Score	Description
Bowels	0	Incontinent (or needs to be given enemas)
	1	Occasional accident (once a week)
	2	Continent
Bladder	0	Incontinent or catheterized or unable to manage alone
	1	Occasional accident (maximum once per 24 hours)
	2	Continent
Grooming	0	Needs help with personal care
	1	Independent face/hair/teeth/shaving
Toilet use	0	Dependent
	1	Needs some help but could do something alone
	2	Independent (on and off, dressing, wiping)
Feeding	0	Unable
	1	Needs help with cutting, spreading butter etc.
	2	Independent
Transfers	0	Unable, no sitting balance
	1	Major help from one or two people, can sit
	2	Minor help (verbal or physical)
	3	Independent
Mobility	0	Immobile
	1	Wheelchair independent, including corners
	2	Walks with help of one person (verbal or physical)
	3	Independent but may use any aid
Dressing	0	Dependent
	1	Needs help but can do half unaided
	2	Independent including buttons, zips, laces etc.
Stairs	0	Unable
	1	Needs help (verbal, physical)
	2	Independent
Bathing	0	Dependent
		Independent or in shower

easily identified. Rehabilitation units in the UK are gaining experience with this measure and it has become one of a basket of measures undertaken.

Other ADL measures include the Nottingham extended ADL scale, which goes beyond personal care to include domestic and household management activities. This was originally used for stroke patients living in the community, it includes specific areas for mobility, kitchen, domestic, and leisure pursuits and is shown in Table 5.5.

Handicap

The handicap dimensions in the original WHO ICIDH text refer to orientation, physical independence, mobility, occupation, social integration, and economic self-sufficiency. Several scales have been derived, of which the London Handicap Scale and the Edinburgh Rehabilitation Status Scale have become best known. Social integration is a measure of a person's behaviour and therefore, in the absence of mental illness or a personality disorder, it is a useful measure of social function. The Frenchay Activities Index also describes this aspect of life. Well-being is difficult to measure in either health or social settings and many profiles have been devised to identify subjective views on how well people feel and how satisfied they are with life. The Sickness Impact Profile and the SF36 are two which have been recommended, and the latter has been used widely in patients with musculoskeletal problems. It is probably the preferred global index of health status, which complements indices of disability rather than being useful as a single tool. It is not particularly good in some situations, for instance in people with stroke and traumatic brain injury living in the community. The Nottingham Health Profile has been developed to measure the way that health problems affect normal activities and responses to the questionnaire are weighted. Refinements of this profile are continually being made.

Conclusions

This chapter shows the complexity of the whole subject. Doctors in training are often confused by what scales to use

Table 5.5 Nottingham Extended ADL Index

Activity	Questions (Do you…?)	Not at all	With help	Alone, with difficulty	Alone, easily
Mobility	Walk around outside?				
	Climb stairs?				
	Get in and out of the car?				
	Walk over uneven ground?				
	Cross roads?				
	Travel on public transport?				
Kitchen	Manage to feed yourself?				
	Manage to make yourself a hot drink?				
	Take hot drinks from one room to another?				
	Do the washing-up?				
	Make yourself a hot snack?				
Domestic tasks	Manage your own money when you are out?				
	Wash small items of clothing?				
	Do a full clothes wash?				
Leisure activities	Read newspapers or books?				
	Use the telephone?				
	Write letters?				
	Go out socially?				
	Manage your own garden?				
	Drive a car?				

Scoring: 0 = not at all–with help; 1 = alone with difficulty–alone easily.

and the following are a selection of measures with which most clinicians should be familiar and should use when treating disabled people in acute and in rehabilitation settings.

- Medical Research Council (MRC) Grades of Muscle Testing
- Motricity Index
- Grip strength
- Nine-hole peg test
- 10 metre timed walk test/6 minutes walk test
- Modified Barthel ADL Index
- Nottingham Extended ADL Index
- Hodkinson's Mental Test
- Modified Ashworth Scale in spasticity.

In addition, the London Handicap Scale and SF36 are worth knowing within the context of a rehabilitation unit.

Reference

1. Bohannon, R. W. and Smith, M. B. (1986). Inter rates reliability of a Modified Ashworth Scale of muscle spasticity. *Physical Therapy*, **67**, 206–7.

Further reading

Wade, D. T. (ed.) (1992). *Measurement in neurological rehabilitation.* Oxford University Press, Oxford.

Section B

The management of physical disabilities

6

Spasticity

Introduction

Spasticity is probably the most common management challenge in the field of neurological rehabilitation. Poorly treated spasticity can lead to joint contracture, pain, unnecessary disability, and problems maintaining suitable postures for feeding, communication, and other aspects of daily living (Fig. 6.1). The proper treatment of spasticity can often have major benefit for the overall quality of life and is one of the more rewarding challenges for the rehabilitation physician.

What is spasticity?

Spasticity can be described as a motor disorder characterized by a velocity-dependent increase in tonic stretch reflexes with exaggerated tendon jerks. This is usually caused by any process in the brain or spinal cord that reduces or destroys the inhibitory neural influence on the spinal reflex arc. It is usually accompanied by impairment of voluntary muscle activation which in turn can cause weakness and clumsiness of voluntary movement. The range of voluntary movement is often reduced to a small number of stereotyped patterns referred to as 'spastic

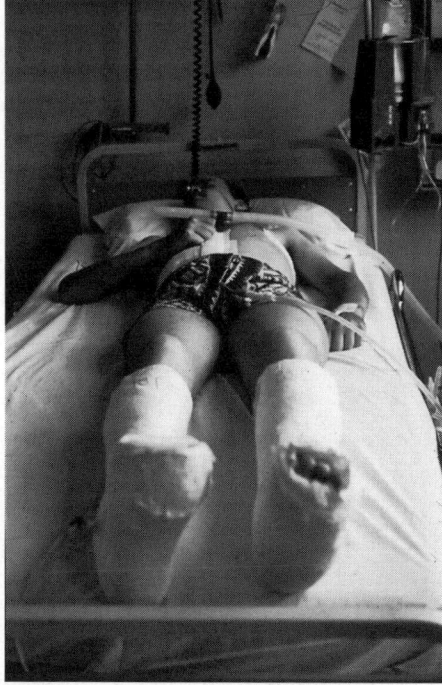

Fig. 6.1 The problems of badly treated spasticity—joint contracture, pain, problems with feeding, dressing and communication.

synergies'. Clinically it is classically demonstrated by imposing a passive movement on the limb which induces an involuntary activation of the stretched muscle. Response is usually velocity dependent, being larger in response to rapid stretch than slow stretch. Sometimes such passive movement can trigger a 'spasm'—an involuntary co-activation of agonist and antagonist muscles of one or more limbs which is often painful. In susceptible individuals such spasms are often triggered by minimal cutaneous stimulation and can be a major disability for the individual. Sometimes, particularly in lower limb extensor muscles, a characteristic pattern of response is seen known as the 'clasp knife response'—when the muscle is stretched progressively, its initial response is the usual velocity-sensitive resistance, but once a certain length is achieved the resistance dies away and the extensor muscle becomes relatively flaccid.

It is important to emphasize that spasticity is essentially a dynamic phenomenon. Although it can be demonstrated on bedside testing, the severity, distribution, and functional consequence of the spasticity can vary quite dramatically in different positions and will also vary over time according to such unpredictable factors as fatigue, stress, external irritants such as clothing, catheter leg bags or orthoses, or in response to different medications. Assessment over a prolonged period of observation is sometimes necessary for adequate management.

Goals and outcomes

The treatment of spasticity, like all rehabilitation processes, should start with the establishment of specific achievable goals and a carefully planned strategy to achieve those goals. The first consideration is often whether it is necessary to treat the spasticity at all. Spasticity can be useful for the individual. For example, spasticity in a leg may serve as a brace to support weight whilst transferring or walking. Arm spasms can occasionally be useful in assisting dressing. It is also worth considering some of the significant side effects of treatment, particularly the oral anti-spastic agents. These can easily induce weakness and fatigue which overall can be more detrimental than leaving the spasticity untreated. However, in general terms there are three aims of treatment:
• to improve function
• to reduce the risk of unnecessary complication
• to alleviate pain.
Occasionally an aim is not specifically to help the patient but to ease nursing care and to assist with the maintenance of hygiene, dressing, and transferring in order to ease the workload of the main carer or nursing staff.

Once the goal has been established then a suitable outcome measure should be chosen that will help to determine whether that goal has been achieved. Unfortunately there are few documented reliable measures of spasticity. The few available tend to be measures of impairment and not measures of disability and handicap. The best known is the

Modified Ashworth Scale (see Chapter 5). There are other biomechanical or neurophysiological techniques that can quantify spasticity but most of these are not practical in the clinical setting. A clinical goal should have an appropriate clinical outcome measure. For example, if the aim of treatment is to reduce pain then a pain scale should be used as the monitoring agent. If a specific functional improvement is required then an appropriate functional or disability scale should be used (see Chapter 5).

An approach to treatment

Alleviating exacerbating factors

Spasticity should be seen as a problem that has a number of underlying causes. It is particularly important for people who are comatose, cognitively impaired, or unable to communicate. Common causes include urinary retention or infection, severe constipation, skin irritation such as pressure sores or increased sensory stimulus from external causes such as ill-fitting orthotic appliances and catheter leg bags. Sometimes exacerbation of spasticity can indicate an underlying abdominal emergency or lower limb fracture, particularly in those who are unable to appreciate pain and not able to localize their problem.

Positioning and seating

Correct positioning, particularly for the immobile patient, is probably the most important aspect of management. Incorrect positioning in bed can easily, for example, exacerbate extensor spasm and problems are eased simply by sitting the patient upright. It is often a matter of trial and error to find a posture that reduces spasticity. Side lying, sitting, and standing can all be helpful in different circumstances. Proper seating is vital. The fundamental principle is that the body should be maintained in a balanced, symmetrical, and stable posture which is both comfortable and maximizes function. There are many different types of seating system but all have the ultimate aim of stabilization of the pelvis without lateral tilt or rotation but with a slight anterior tilt so the spine adopts a normal lumbar lordosis, thoracic kyphosis, and cervical lordosis. The hip is normally maintained at a angle of slightly more than 90° and this is often facilitated by a seat cushion with a slight backward slope. Knees and ankles are normally at 90°. In people with severe spasticity this posture may need a variety of seating adjustments such as foot straps, knee blocks, adductor pommels, lumbar supports, lateral trunk supports, and a variety of head and neck support systems. The input of a physiotherapist and in particular a seating specialist is vital.

Physiotherapy

In addition to the advice on seating and positioning physiotherapists have a variety of other anti-spastic techniques at their disposal. Heat is often used for relaxation of a spastic muscle but unfortunately the effect is often short lived. Cold can also inhibit a spastic muscle but once again the effect is short lived, perhaps only out-lasting the application of the cold by about half an hour. Direct electrical stimulation of the muscle can also be used with an anti-spastic effect that can last several hours. There are a number of different dynamic techniques such as the Bobath, proprioceptive neuromuscular facilitation, the Brunnstrom technique and the approach of Carr and Shepherd which all claim an anti-spastic effect. However, there is little evidence that any particular technique is better than another for the management of spasticity. A consensus is that it is important to put a spastic muscle through a full range of movement in order to try to prevent contracture. There is no agreement on how long a muscle needs to be stretched in order to prevent contracture but some guidelines suggest that muscles should be put at full stretch for at least two hours in each 24 hours. Finally, the physiotherapist can be useful for the application of splints, casts, and orthoses. The range of movement in a contracted limb can definitely be improved by the serial application of splints or -casts—with a new plaster cast being applied every few days as the range of movement improves (Fig. 6.2). A variety of orthoses are now available that can help hold a spastic limb in a neutral or functional position and minimize the risk of contracture. Figure 6.3 illustrates a simple ankle foot orthosis that can be useful particularly in a plantar flexed and inverted spastic foot.

Oral medication

Pharmacological management for spasticity is not usually an important component in the overall treatment regime. Although there are now four available anti-spastic agents all suffer from a range of troublesome side effects, particularly weakness and fatigue. Paradoxically oral drugs are probably most use in mild to moderate cases when lower doses can have a desirable effect. In more severe cases when higher doses are needed the anti-spastic effects are often of minimal benefit and negated by unacceptable

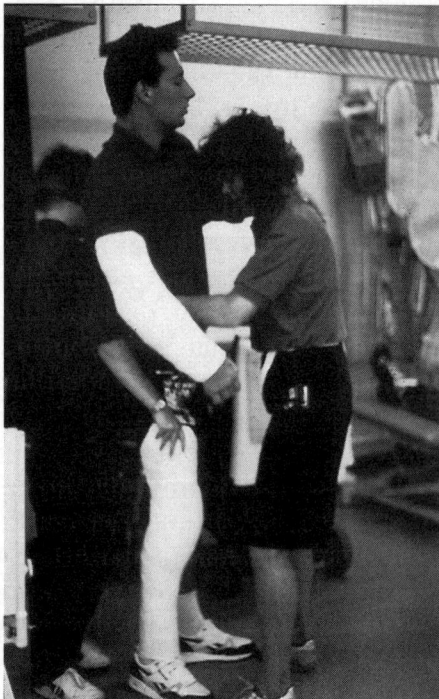

Fig. 6.2 Serial casting.

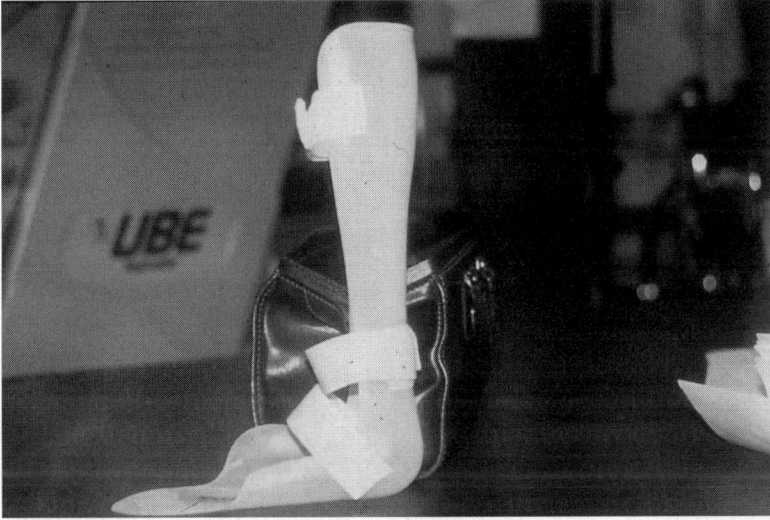

Fig. 6.3 Ankle foot orthosis.

weakness and drowsiness. The four available drugs are listed below.

Diazepam
This was the first anti-spastic agent to be used and probably has an anti-spastic effect by facilitating GABA-mediated inhibition. It does this by increasing affinity of GABA receptors for the indigenous neurotransmitter, thus enhancing pre-synaptic inhibition. However, it is rarely used in clinical practice as it induces profound drowsiness and weakness at effective anti-spastic doses.

Baclofen
Baclofen is a GABA B receptor agonist but probably also has a pre-synaptic inhibitory effect on the release of excitatory neurotransmitters such as glutamate, aspartate, and substance P. It probably acts at a spinal cord level by inhibition of polysynaptic spinal reflexes. It is a useful and effective anti-spastic agent but once again is limited by side effects of drowsiness, fatigue, and muscle weakness. It has a short half-life and each dose lasts only 3–4 hours. There is little benefit beyond a dosage of 80 mg daily.

....

Dantrolene sodium

The mode of action of dantrolene is directly on skeletal muscle and it appears to suppress the release of calcium from the cytoplasmic reticulum with the consequent inhibition of excitation, contraction, and coupling. It can be effective but is often limited by drowsiness, dizziness, weakness, fatigue, and diarrhoea and has the additional problem of liver toxicity.

Tizanidine

This is an agent that has been available in Europe for some years but has recently been licensed in the UK. The mode of action probably arises from agonist activity at noradrenergic alpha 2 receptors which results in direct impairment of excitatory amino acid release from spinal neurons and concomitant inhibition of facilitatory caerulo-spinal pathways. It has a similar anti-spastic effect to baclofen but does seem to produce less clinical weakness and, with more experience, could be the most clinically useful and effective anti-spastic agent.

A number of other drugs have been tried including clonidine, L-dopa, glycine, L-threonine, and cannabis but none have yet found a place in clinical practice.

Peripheral treatment

Most spasticity is focal, affecting one or a few muscle groups. The problem with oral therapy is that it will have a generalized systemic effect whereas the aim of treatment is to have an anti-spastic effect only on spastic muscles whilst minimizing side effects. Thus, peripheral techniques have been developed to treat focal spasticity.

Phenol/alcohol nerve blocks and botulinum toxin

It is a relatively simple procedure to identify a peripheral nerve by means of a needle electrode. The tip of the needle is manipulated until it is as close as possible to the nerve and then a small volume of phenol or alcohol can be injected down the same needle. This will usually produce an immediate nerve block with consequent relaxation of the supplied muscle. Any accessible peripheral nerve can be blocked in this way and the most useful are the obturator nerve (for adductor spasticity) (Fig. 6.4), the posterior tibial nerve (for calf spasticity), the sciatic nerve (for hamstring spasticity), and sometimes the median, ulnar, and musculo-cutaneous nerves of the arm (for flexor arm spasticity). A block will usually last 2–3 months although permanent effects can sometimes occur. If the nerve blocked is a mixed motor sensory nerve then there can be troublesome sensory side effects including painful dysaesthesiae.

The technique is effective but often time-consuming and somewhat uncomfortable for the patient. More recently botulinum toxin has been used to directly relax spastic muscles. Botulinum toxin is a potent neurotoxin that blocks the release of acetyl choline from nerve endings. It is now the treatment of first choice for focal dystonias and is finding an increasingly useful place for the management of spasticity. The toxin is diluted in normal saline and injected directly into the spastic muscle. Relaxation is normally induced over a period of a few days and lasts around 2–3 months. The technique is quick, simple, and effective with

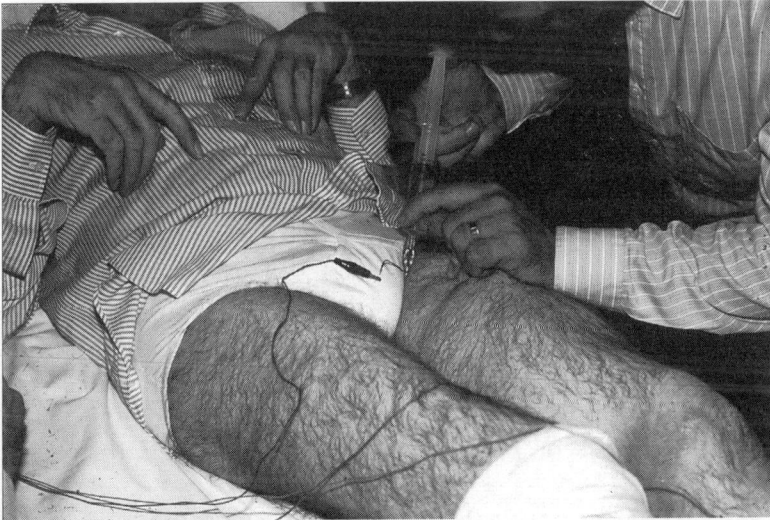

Fig. 6.4 Injection of the obturator nerve with phenol.

virtually no reported side effects. Occasionally a flu-like illness can occur for a few days or there can be problems of over-relaxation of the muscle inducing unnecessary weakness. However, the toxin is expensive and thus unlikely to be used in countries where resources are scarce.

Intrathecal techniques
The use of intrathecal baclofen was first described in 1984. This technique usually involves the implantation of a subcutaneous pump to allow programmable intrathecal delivery of baclofen through a silastic catheter. There is no doubt that this is a useful technique in more severe and resistant spasticity. However, there are obvious disadvantages to a surgical procedure, particularly in severely disabled people and an additional risk of technical problems including failure of the pump or catheter movement. Occasionally in people who have no motor, sensory, bowel, or bladder function then intrathecal phenol can be used in the lumbar spine to destroy the peripheral nerves in the cauda equina. This is a dramatic technique but for those who are already paraplegic and incontinent it can be useful, particularly to relieve painful spasticity and to facilitate nursing care.

Surgical and orthopaedic procedures
There is rarely need to resort to surgery for the management of spasticity except in the occasional severe or resistant case or for the management of fixed contractures. However, a few techniques are still used. Anterior and posterior rhizotomy have been performed for many years and more refined surgery is now possible including microsurgical lesion of the dorsal root entry zone (DREZotomy). A less invasive technique of percutaneous radiofrequency rhizotomy is also sometimes helpful. Spinal cord and cerebellar stimulation has been reported to be effective but the effects tend to be relatively weak and short lived with the additional risk of problems with equipment failure and expense.

Occasionally surgical repositioning of joints and limbs can facilitate proper seating and ease positioning and the application of orthoses. One of the more common orthopaedic interventions is an Achilles' tendon lengthening procedure for fixed equinus deformity. Severe adductor spasticity can sometimes be helped by obturator neurectomy or adductor tenotomy. Surgery in the upper limb is not generally successful, but various tenotomy and tendon lengthening procedures are possible, including lengthening of the biceps and brachioradialis, lengthening of the flexor carpi ulnaris and flexor carpi radialis for wrist flexor spasticity and transfer of the flexor pollicis longus to the radial site of the thumb for isolated thumb-in-palm deformities.

Conclusions

The management of spasticity is complicated. Most people can be managed by a combination of physiotherapy and local nerve block or botulinum injection sometimes combined with relatively low-dose oral medication. The use of more advanced intrathecal and surgical procedures is rarely needed unless complications have arisen, often due to inappropriate early management. Spasticity requires the input of a full rehabilitation team involving in particular the physician, orthotist, and physiotherapist. The management of spasticity can often give rewarding results and lead to major improvements in the quality of life.

Further reading

Barnes, M. P. (1998). The management of spasticity. *Age and Ageing*, **27**, 239–45.

Barnes, M. P., McLellan, D. L., and Sutton, R. (1993). Spasticity. In: Greenwood, R., Barnes, M. P., McMillan, T. M., and Ward, C. D. (ed.) *Neurological rehabilitation*, pp.161–72. Churchill Livingstone, London.

Ko Ko, C.and Ward, A. B. (1997). The management of spasticity. *British Journal of Hospital Medicine*, **19**, 400–5.

Skeil, D. A. and Barnes, M. P. (1994). The local treatment of spasticity. *Clinical Rehabilitation*, **8**, 240–6.

7

....

Continence

Neural control of bladder function extends from the frontal lobes to the sacral cord and thus it is not surprising that bladder dysfunction is extremely common in neurological disease and trauma. Incontinence is a major disabling problem but can often be greatly assisted, usually by fairly simple means. Two major goals of treatment need to be borne in mind. One goal is the management of symptoms, particularly incontinence. However, a second and vital goal is to minimize the risks to kidney function. Until recently the leading cause of death in spinal cord injury was renal failure. Such death is almost invariably preventable by proper rehabilitation and urological assessment and by close follow-up. Nowadays renal compromise and death would normally indicate inadequate care rather than an inevitable conclusion.

Normal bladder function

Anatomy and physiology of the urinary system is complicated and not fully understood. However, a simple overview of basic anatomy and neural control of bladder function is possible and will allow practical and effective measures to be initiated (Fig. 7.1).

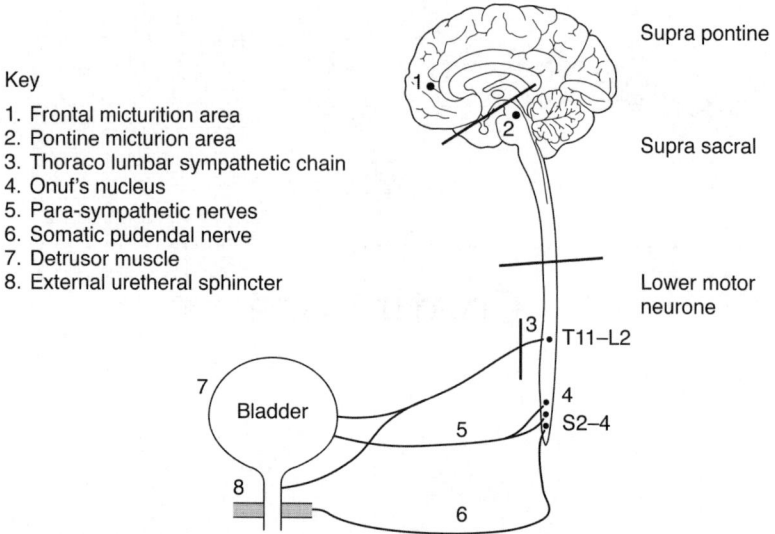

Key

1. Frontal micturition area
2. Pontine micturion area
3. Thoraco lumbar sympathetic chain
4. Onuf's nucleus
5. Para-sympathetic nerves
6. Somatic pudendal nerve
7. Detrusor muscle
8. External uretheral sphincter

Supra pontine

Supra sacral

Lower motor
neurone

T11–L2

S2–4

Bladder

Fig. 7.1   Overview of neural control of bladder function.

The bladder is composed of the detrusor muscle that allows urine to be collected and the bladder to expand without a rise in pressure, until voiding is imminent. This phenomenon is described as compliance. When voiding is started, the bladder smooth muscle will contract. At the same time the external urethral sphincter will need to relax. This sphincter is composed of striated muscle fibres with separate innervation from the rest of the detrusor.

Neural innervation of the bladder and sphincter

Parasympathetic and sympathetic nerves

The main nerve supply to the body of detrusor smooth muscle is from parasympathetic neurons lying in the cord at the S2/3/4 level. The bladder, particularly the neck, also receives a nerve supply from the thoracolumbar sympathetic chain. In man the role of the sympathetic innervation is not entirely clear. The post-ganglionic sympathetic fibres are noradrenergic whereas the pre-ganglionic sympathetic fibres and the parasympathetic fibres are cholinergic. This classification is useful for management purposes but is probably an over-simplification and it is now known that other neurotransmitters and neuromodulators have a complicated and ill-understood role at sympathetic and parasympathetic terminals.

Somatic nerves

The striated muscle of the urethral sphincter has motor innervation by a discrete nucleus (Onuf's nucleus) lying at the S2/3/4 level in the spinal cord. The cells are integrated with the parasympathetic supply which also arises in this vicinity. The motor fibres pass from the S2/3/4 nerve roots into the pudendal nerve which branches to both the urethral sphincter and anal sphincter.

Sensory nerves

Sensation of bladder fullness is in man mostly conveyed through the pelvic and pudendal nerves to the spinal cord and upwards via the lateral-spinothalamic tract. Afferent fibres will synapse in Onuf's nucleus to form a simple spinal reflex as well as also synapsing with the sympathetic chain.

Pontine micturition centre

The centre in the pons appears to have a coordinating influence regulating long spinal reflexes on the one hand whilst receiving modulatory, usually inhibitory, influences from higher brain centres on the other hand.

Higher cortical influence

It is known that the frontal lobes have an influence on micturition. Pathology in the anterio-medial parts of the frontal lobe can produce a variety of problems including urgency, urge incontinence, loss of bladder sensation, or urinary retention. Lesions in other parts of the frontal lobes can produce social disinhibition and voiding at inappropriate times and places, although in such circumstances the actual voiding mechanism is usually normal.

Pathophysiology

Although the neural control of bladder function is complex there are basically only three types of bladder disorder according to the level of interruption of the neural pathway—suprapontine, suprasacral, and lower motor neuron.

Lesion above the pons micturition centre

The activity of the pontine micturition centre is modulated from higher centres mainly by inhibitory input, particularly from the frontal lobes but also the basal ganglia and other centres. Disconnection from above, such as by frontal lobe damage, periventricular demyelination in multiple sclerosis, disorders of the basal ganglia, and dilatation of the anterior horns of the lateral ventricles in hydrocephalus, all tend to result in hyperreflexic bladder contractions. However, rarely the opposite can be true and urinary retention can result following the failure of initiation of voluntary micturition.

Lesion between the pontine micturition centre and the sacral spinal cord

The descending pathways between the pontine centre and the sacral cord tend to be inhibitory and thus a lesion in the tract will tend to result in a hyperreflexic bladder. This means that bladder contraction is stimulated by a small amount of urine and will usually be associated with the symptoms of urgency, frequency, and sometimes urge incontinence.

The descending tracts, however, are also responsible for coordination between the external sphincter and detrusor. Thus a lesion in the cord can also be responsible for failure of this coordination mechanism resulting in 'detrusor sphincter dyssynergia'. This means that the sphincter will fail to relax appropriately when the detrusor contracts. This can be dangerous as it will lead to high intravesical pressure leading to back pressure on the kidneys and upper tract dilatation. In terms of symptoms it usually results in interrupted bursts of urinary flow depending on the pressure differentials between the forces in the detrusor tending to expel urine and the forces in the sphincter tending to retain urine.

Other problems are possible. In some people hyperreflexic contractions occur but these are poorly sustained and the bladder only empties incompletely. This can give rise to increased post-micturition residual volumes, particularly if there is some degree of dyssynergia.

Lower motor neuron lesions

Damage to the sacral nerves S2/3/4 will usually result in a lower motor neuron defect of bladder function and a loss of bladder sensation. Involuntary initiation of micturition is absent or reduced and the bladder will tend to become hypotonic and non-compliant. The external sphincter will be relaxed although often there is some residual control on the bladder neck because of the elastic nature of the tissues. Stress incontinence will tend to be common as urine will leak with a sudden rise in intra-abdominal (and hence intravesical) pressure during straining, coughing, or sneezing. Higher residual urine volume is also possible due to the impaired detrusor contraction.

Overall the level of the lesion may act as a guide to underlying pathophysiology. However, there are many exceptions to these guidelines and it would be unwise and potentially dangerous to rely on the level of the lesion as an absolute indicator of underlying problem. Symptoms are also a poor guide to pathophysiology. Table 7.1 indicates some of the underlying causes of the commonest urinary symptoms.

Management of urinary problems

The primary task is to determine the nature of the underlying problem. There are three principle questions that will need to be answered:
- Is there impairment of renal function?
- Is there a failure of bladder emptying?
- Is there detrusor hyperreflexia?

Table 7.1 Underlying causes of urinary symptoms. (After Fowler and Fowler (1993).)

Urgency and frequency
  Detrusor hyperreflexia
  Detrusor instability
  Retention
  Impaired detrusor contraction
  Impaired sphincter relaxation
  Detrusor sphincter dyssynergia
  Failure to initiate micturition reflex or local urological causes
    (e.g. prostatic hypertrophy)

Incontinence
  Detrusor hyperreflexia
  Detrusor instability
  Retention with overflow
  Stress incontinence

Is there impairment of renal function?

Screening of the upper urinary tract is important if there are any urinary symptoms. Indeed in some people routine screening of the upper tract even in the absence of symptoms is necessary, such as in those with spinal cord injury. An intravenous urogram and a simple biochemical test such as serum creatinine will answer this basic question. If these are normal then follow-up of individuals at risk can usually be by serial biochemical screening and non-invasive ultrasound to detect any upper tract dilatation.

Is there a failure of bladder emptying?

Post-micturition urine volume can be obtained by catheterization and an approximation obtained from an ultrasound scan of the bladder. This is usually sufficient to establish whether emptying is impaired. Residual urine greater than 100 ml is a generally accepted level at which intervention is necessary. Residual urine can pre-dispose to infection, stone formation, and can contribute to impairment of renal function, particularly if the failure to empty is associated with a high intravesical pressure and back pressure up the ureters to the kidney.

Occasionally failure to empty can be managed by artificial stimulation—by suprapubic tapping or perianal stimulation. Sometimes manual compression of the bladder by suprapubic pressure (Credé's manoeuvre) can raise the intravesical pressure sufficiently to empty the bladder, particularly in those who have some degree of sphincter weakness. However, these emptying procedures will need to be preceded by a cystometrogram. There is no point in stimulating bladder emptying if at the same time there is back pressure and a risk of damage to the upper urinary tract.

In most cases failure of bladder emptying will require mechanical drainage. The most useful method is intermittent clean self catheterization. Intermittent catheterization is carried out by the person or sometimes by a carer about four or five times in every 24 hours. In this way volumes are kept less than about 500 ml on each occasion. The technique is not sterile but clean using an 8F or 10F plastic catheter. The technique can eventually be taught to the great majority of people though obviously a period of training, usually by a continence nurse advisor, is necessary. The technique is best suited to those with a good capacity bladder as well as a well innervated sphincter and thus people who are able to retain a reasonable volume without leakage in between catheterizations. There is a slight risk of bladder infection but this is minimal.

Occasionally intermittent self-catheterization is not possible or the type of problem makes it undesirable. In such cases residual urine will need draining by an indwelling catheter. A silastic catheter should be used (14–18F in an adult) with a small balloon retainer, preferably no more than 5 ml. Unfortunately there are many complications of catheterization including leakage, blockage, stone formation, and particularly infection. It is a common fault to counteract leakage by inserting a larger catheter. This will usually just increase detrusor irritability and the urethra becomes more patulous. If catheter expulsion is a problem sometimes a trial of anti-cholinergic medication can be used to suppress detrusor activity. However, it is now becoming more common to use suprapubic catheterization in the long term and this can prevent recurrent problems of catheter insertion and the risks of urethral trauma and stricture but will still share the same problems of infection, stone formation, and leakage.

Very occasionally retention due to poor detrusor contraction can be assisted by the use of cholinergic or anticholinesterase medication. Selected α-1 blockers such as Alfuzosin and Prazosin can also be used as an adjunct to symptomatic treatment of a urinary obstruction caused by benign prostatic hypertrophy. It should also be remembered that prostatic hypertrophy and other local neurological causes can exacerbate an underlying neuro-urological problem.

Is there detrusor hyperreflexia?

The symptoms of urinary frequency, urgency, and urge incontinence will often indicate detrusor hyperreflexia but the only satisfactory way of confirming this problem is by cystometrography. This is a very straightforward technique. It involves the passage of two small catheters into the bladder. One is used for filling the bladder with fluid whilst the other monitors the pressure. Usually a further catheter is introduced above the rectum in order to measure fluctuation in intra-abdominal pressure which will be reflected in raised intravesical pressure. The rectal pressure is deducted from the intravesical pressure in order to get a true measure of bladder pressure. The bladder is filled and voiding patterns can be monitored. Sometimes radio-opaque fluid is used to fill the bladder which, with radio-logical screening, can allow a more accurate determination of urine filling and voiding.

The management of detrusor hyperreflexia is in most people fairly straightforward. A small number can control more minor problems by a rigid bladder drill including emptying of the bladder at frequent and regular intervals. However, most people will need some form of oral medication to reduce bladder contractions. Anti-cholinergic medication is the most effective and Oxybutinin is the most commonly used agent. There are problems of unwanted anticholinergic side effects including dry mouth, constipation, and blurring of vision but generally the drug is reasonably well tolerated. Alternative, although less satisfactory, agents are Propantheline and Imipramine. In some cases urgency and urge incontinence can continue despite anti-cholinergic medication and in such people, and in those with stress incontinence, then protection against the embarrassment of leakage is necessary. In men condom drainage is usually satisfactory. In men who cannot satisfactorily wear a condom and for women there are a variety of absorbent pads that can be worn. The pads may also be useful for some people with persistent catheter leakage and many individuals prefer the additional security of pads to prevent embarrassment. Advice from a specially trained nurse continence advisor can be invaluable at this stage.

Surgical management

A number of surgical techniques are possible for the important minority of people who are not adequately managed by the simpler measures outlined above. Obviously at this point urological advice and expertise will be required. It is not possible to go into much detail about surgical procedures in this book but a few of the commoner techniques will be mentioned.

Sphincter ablation

An alternative to indwelling catheterization in the male is sphincter ablation followed by condom drainage. Another option is an indwelling endourethral stent which effectively produces a mechanical bypass to the sphincter. The intrasphincter use of botulinum toxin has also recently been tried with some success in order to relax the external sphincter.

Urinary diversions

If straightforward methods of draining the bladder via a urethral or suprapubic catheter fail then other forms of urinary diversion are possible. An intestinal conduit can be a fashioned from the bladder to the skin (the Metrofanoff procedure). However, the conduit will still require intermittent catheterization. Continent urostomies can be provided while the ureter can be redirected into a ileal loop which will drain into a stoma bag.

Other procedures

Intractable hyperreflexic bladders can now be replaced by bowel segments which in turn can be emptied by intermittent self-catheterization. In a similar technique segments of ileum can be laid into the bladder wall to augment capacity and absorb rises in intravesical pressure. This is the so-called 'clam cystoplasty'. Artificial urethral sphincters can now also be inserted. More recently individuals, particularly those with spinal cord injury, have been implanted with anterior sacral root stimulators. These are activated by a radio receiver and the sacral roots stimulated, resulting in detrusor contraction.

Conclusions

Incontinence and other urinary symptoms are very common in neurological disabling disorders. Incontinence can be a major disability and handicap but effective management is usually straightforward and can result in a major improvement in the quality of life for many people. Most people with urinary problems can be helped and death from renal involvement should now be extremely rare. Every rehabilitation team should have the ability to initiate simple symptomatic treatments and should have ready access to a nurse continence advisor and urological specialists.

Further reading

Fowler, C. J. and Fowler, C. G. (1993). Neurogenic bladder dysfunction and its management. In: Greenwood, R., Barnes, M. P., McMillan, T. M., and Ward, C. D. (ed.) *Neurological rehabilitation*, pp.269–77. Churchill Livingstone, London.

Gelber, D. A. (1994). Bladder dysfunction. In: Good, D. C. and Couch, J. R. (ed.) *Handbook of neurorehabilitation*, pp.373–402. Marcel Dekker, New York.

Parsons, K. F., Feneley, R. C. L., and Torrens, M. J. (1994). Rehabilitation and management of neuropathic bladder. In: Illis, L. S. (ed.) *Neurological rehabilitation*, (2nd Edn), pp.349–81. Blackwell Scientific, London.

Roe, B. (1992). *Clinical nursing practice. The promotion and management of continence*. Prentice Hall, London.

Rushton, D. N. (1994). *Handbook of neuro-urology*. Marcel Dekker, New York.

8

....

Sex and sexuality

The most ignored and least discussed of disability issues is sex and sexuality. Professionals are often very embarrassed to talk about the subject and many still display the attitude of thinking that it is not relevant to the lives of disabled people and not worth discussing. Disabled people are like everybody else and have the same sexual urges and feelings as the rest of the population. The importance of sex and sexuality and discussing the emotional needs of disabled individuals and their families and carers is thus an essential part of discovering the personality requesting help. Sexual function taken outside the context of emotional needs is really very straightforward and concentrates on physical function. Sexuality on the other hand includes making relationships, the whole question of self-esteem, personal appearance, and attraction to potential partners and is the very essence of the human spirit. It plays a full part in the lives of not only disabled people, but of the general population as well.

The desires and wishes for emotional and personal attachments of disabled people are no different from those of the rest of the population. They are often played down, and it is known that people who have been disabled either congenitally or from a very early age have decreased expectations. Their families also have decreased expectations and it is perhaps not surprising that many disabled people are scared or embarrassed to raise sex and sexuality as an issue. It is therefore important for the doctor or other members of the rehabilitation team to bring up the subject in an open and frank way, so that the whole subject can be discussed freely. It is often found that there is a huge relief of emotional frustration once a disabled person can find an appropriate outlet for their feelings. Psychosexual clinics are appearing, but are still relatively rare. The teaching of sex and sexuality is now part of the curriculum for specialist trainees in rehabilitation medicine and concentrates on both the psychosocial aspects and the physical function. Various techniques can get round the physical problems and some will be mentioned below. However, the whole idea of a man or woman with a physical disability discussing their sex life with a total stranger fills many with dread. For instance, how might they be able to carry out intercourse while having a catheter *in situ*. Will they have an episode of incontinence during intercourse, how will they physically get close enough to each other, and how might they relate a relationship to their friends and family? How will they deal with the prospect perhaps of pregnancy and parenthood? Disabled people may well fail initially (just like most of the able-bodied population) but will need to persevere, to learn how to be intimate with their partners, without being overwhelmed by failing to match up to their own expectations.

Sexuality

While sex is the act of intimacy, sexuality is the persona of the individual which attracts potential partners. One's ability to be a part of society and to be recognized as a person with a contribution to society is a strong catalyst to developing the necessary assertiveness to express sexuality. In order to meet people with whom one would wish to develop friendships and relationships, one must first be able to function and to use the standard facilities whereby people get together. This usually includes being able to communicate, to get out of the house, to have the financial means to socialize, get to college, work, or a day centre, etc., have the cognitive and personality skills to attract people and very often the transport to be flexible and available. As stated above, disabled people often have to cope with considerable disadvantages, such as low esteem from their appearance in a wheelchair, lack of confidence about what people may think of them, particularly if they are incontinent or wear a catheter, and young people may be actively hindered by their families in expressing their own sexual feelings. Many men may be impotent and 80 to 90 per cent of these are usually psychogenic. With time, relaxation, and confidence, impotence usually resolves, but there are always going to be a few who are going to need help to get over this problem. Again, as stated above, sexual performance need not necessarily be considered as the only yardstick to measure satisfaction in personal relationships. The promotion of quality of life in an open and full relationship may be just as rewarding as the ability to carry out sexual intercourse.

Male sexual function

Impotence tends to be associated with lesions of the spinal cord or cauda equina. Involvement of the autonomic and sensory pathways may give rise to impaired erectile function in males, due to impaired vasocongestion of the corpora cavernosa and spongiosa. The lower the level of the lesion, the more likely that impotence will be organic in nature. Those people with an intact sacral portion of the spinal cord are likely to achieve reflex erection, although this may be inadequate for intercourse. Overall, about half of spinal cord injured men have sufficient erection for intercourse. Sacral anterior stimulator implants can be used to achieve erection, but more commonly, men with erectile dysfunction can be managed by the use of intra-cavernosal injections of Papaverine. This can give rise to penile fibrosis, but the technique is certainly successful. Prostaglandins E1 is again of interest in producing penile rigidity. More recently, Sildenafil (Viagra) has become available. This acts as a selective inhibitor of the phosphodiesterase isoenzyme PDE5 and prolongs cGMP activity in erectile tissue. It thus amplifies the natural vasodilatatory actions of nitric oxide, thereby enhancing the erectile response to sexual stimulation. Its normal dosage ranges from 50–100 mg to produce a response, but further reading is recommended in the British National Formulary. It is expensive and its prescription has remained restricted in the NHS.

Ejaculatory function is affected more commonly than erectile function in spinal cord injured men. Only 5 per cent of men with a complete upper motor neurone lesion and 18 per cent with a complete lower motor neurone lesion report any persistence of the ability to achieve ejaculation. The treatment may consist of vibration applied to the penis with or without electrical stimulation, using a probe placed in the rectum. This can promote ejaculation by allowing the semen to be collected, but it has to be stated that these techniques are in the management of infertility in spinal cord injured patients rather than in the promotion of the sexual act. Electro-ejaculation is also possible in the clinic, but again this is for achievement of fertility. All vibration techniques are able to be used at home, but care is required in patients with an injury above the level of D6. Autonomic hyperreflexia can occur with all its attendant problems. Management of urinary infections is obviously important as they will limit already impaired spermatogenesis. Similarly, older fashioned techniques of sphincterotomies may result in retrograde ejaculation of semen and this procedure is finding less and less favour for many other reasons.

Female fertility

One of the main aspects of sexuality in disabled women is that they may not have received education on contraception. While 75 per cent of men report sexual dysfunction, it is less common in women at 56 per cent. However, many describe fatigue, diminished sensation, loss of libido, and orgasmic dysfunction. This is particularly evident in multiple sclerosis and traumatic brain injury. Hyposexuality is a common change after the latter, although disinhibition and hypersexuality have been reported following a frontal injury.

Pregnancy carries with it increased risks, particularly of pressure sores and sepsis, particularly in the urinary tract. Ante-natal care should be carried out in conjunction with a spinal injuries unit. Women with injuries at the D10 level or above are at risk of premature delivery and at D6 and above, of autonomic dysreflexia which is particularly evident as a warning of impending labour. Epidural anaesthesia should be considered as the method of choice for these particular women.

Conclusions

It is not actually known how many people report sexual dysfunction among the disabled population, but figures as high as 72 per cent have been suggested. The importance of counselling, education, and explanation is thus highly desirable and the first step in this process can be for doctors, no matter what their background, to bring the subject up as a routine activity during their assessment of patients and then to refer to the appropriate rehabilitation service. Sexual matters are no less important than any other aspect of one's personal life and they should be given equal consideration in assessing the needs of disabled people.

Further reading

Bancroft, J. (1989). *Human sexuality and its problems.* Churchill Livingstone, Edinburgh.

Bancroft, J. (1993). Impact of environment, stress, occupational and other hazards on sexuality and sexual behaviour. *Environmental Health Perspectives (Supplements)*, **101**, (2), 101–7.

Lechtenberg, R. and Ohl, D. A. (1994). *Sexual dysfunction.* Lea and Febiger, Philadelphia.

Spence, S. H. (1991). *Psychosexual therapy. A cognitive-behavioural approach.* Chapman and Hall, London.

9

....

Eating and swallowing disorders

Introduction

Swallowing disorders are common and their recognition is vital. At least half of people after stroke have swallowing disorders and problems with swallowing are equally common after a traumatic head injury, in Parkinson's disease, and in the latter stages of multiple sclerosis and motor neuron disease. A variety of other neurological problems, such as myasthenia gravis and some muscular dystrophies, as well as a range of local pathology, such as mouth and laryngeal cancer, can also cause problems. Sometimes other less obvious pathologies can be responsible, albeit temporarily, for swallowing difficulties such as infections in the mouth, painful ulcers, or painful and poor fitting dentures. Tracheostomy tubes can also disturb the dynamics of swallowing.

It is important to recognize that a swallowing problem exists. Sometimes the problem is obvious and the individual will volunteer a problem with chewing, swallowing, or coughing during or soon after food. However, sometimes the problem is less obvious, particularly in children or those with cognitive impairments. In such individuals recurrent chest infections may give a clue to intermittent aspiration. Weight loss, malnutrition, taking excessive time over food, food residue in the mouth,

....

excessive secretions, wet or hoarse voice after food can all be clues that a swallowing disorder may exist.

Assessment

A problem with eating should be differentiated from a problem associated with the physical act of swallowing. In some people problems with behaviour, mood, or cognition can all interfere with or prevent eating. A person with traumatic brain injury may not wish to cooperate with the main carer. A person after stroke may have severe perceptual or dyspraxic problems thus making them incapable of using plates and cutlery properly. A problem with receptive language may prevent someone from understanding the instructions that 'dinner is ready'. An individual with severe depression may simply not wish to eat. The author has seen a number of people with terminal disability and profound physical problems who are effectively attempting to commit suicide in the only way open to them, by refusing food. Thus, a swallowing assessment cannot be taken out of context from a general assessment of behaviour, mood, cognition, and intellectual function.

Physical assessment should also not be restricted to the act of swallowing. Close examination of the mouth and tongue may reveal a local cause of a swallowing problem such as carcinoma or painful infection. Problems with poor dental hygiene or ill-fitting dentures can similarly lead to problems. Neurological examination of the cranial nerves may also be required. Table 9.1 indicates the rather complex involvement of different cranial nerves at the different stages of swallowing.

Physical assessment

It is important to understand the four stages as problems can occur at any of these stages. The normal swallowing mechanism is outlined in the next section. The only proper way to make an assessment of the swallowing mechanism is by videofluroscopy. This should be available to all

Table 9.1 Involvement of cranial nerves during swallowing

Cranial nerve	Function
V	Muscles of mastication and sensation to the anterior 2/3 of the tongue and buccal cavity
VII	Nerve to supply the orbicularis oris muscle required for lip closure and taste to the anterior 2/3 of the tongue
IX	Taste and sensation to posterior third of the tongue and buccal cavity and sensation to the tonsils, laryngeal mucosa, and soft palate and involvement of gag and cough reflexes
X	Similar to IX but also involved with phonation and vocal cord closure in the larynx and sensation and motility of the oesophagus
XII	Movement of the tongue

specialist rehabilitation centres but may not be widely available to a community team or within a district general hospital. Unfortunately it is the only way to make an accurate swallowing assessment. It is worth emphasizing that the gag reflex is not an assessment of swallowing but is simply an assessment of a cranial nerve reflex arc. The presence or absence of the gag reflex should never be taken to assess the safety of oral feeding. An idea of the overall swallowing mechanism can be obtained by a simple swallow of a small quantity of water. If the water can be swallowed without due difficulty it is likely the swallowing mechanism is intact but again it must be emphasized that this is not a precise test and must be interpreted with caution. Any doubts in this basic assessment should precipitate a referral to an appropriate centre for a more detailed analysis and videofluoroscopy.

A further aspect of physical assessment is reviewing the posture and positioning during eating and swallowing. As far as possible people should be sat upright with the head and spine erect. In some people, for example those with severe kyphoscoliosis, this is not possible and the best compromise position should be attained.

Carer/feeder assessment

Occasionally an apparent eating or swallowing problem is actually a result of difficulty with the main carer or feeder. Time and care in food preparation is often required and often considerable time and effort is needed in the feeding process. A child with cerebral palsy can, for example, often take up to an hour to take an adequate meal. Rushed preparation, feeding, inappropriate attention to posture, and even to the likes and dislikes of the individual can all lead to problems.

Nutritional assessment

An assessment should be made of nutritional state. Body weight and height measurements can lead to a calculation of the surface area to weight ratio. Ideal ratios are known and an assessment can be made of the adequacy of body weight. Total body fat can be estimated by skin fold measurements such as in biceps, triceps, or iliac sites and once again normal parameters are available. An accurate weight record is sometimes the only way of monitoring improvement as a result of treatment, particularly in children or those with cognitive problems.

Normal swallowing mechanism

Swallowing is conveniently divided into four main stages (Fig. 9.1):
1. Stage 1—Oral preparation: At this stage food is bitten, chewed, and masticated and prepared into a bolus. This phase will clearly rely on proper coordination of the lips, tongue, and jaws and will require an adequate quantity of saliva.
2. Stage 2—Oral phase: This stage involves the voluntary transfer of the bolus or fluid towards the pharynx. The tongue plays a major part in this process and will move the food bolus upwards and backwards to contact with the hard palate. When the bolus reaches the anterior faucial arch the reflex swallow is initiated.

3. Stage 3—Pharyngeal phase: This is a reflex stage no longer under voluntary control. This stage will involve a number of important muscular actions:
   (a) Closure of the velo pharynx to prevent food and fluid refluxing into the nose.
   (b) Closure of the larynx to prevent material entering the larynx. This is achieved by laryngeal elevation and anterior movement which also has the effect of stretching and helping to the open the crico-pharyngeal muscle.
   (c) Peristalsis of the pharynx in order to help propel the bolus towards the oesophagus.
   (d) Opening of the cricopharyngeal muscle and passage of the bolus into the oesophagus.
4. Stage 4—Oesophageal phase: This is again an automatic stage involving passage of the bolus from the relaxed upper oesophageal sphincter at the level of the crico-pharyngeal muscle down the oesophagus to enter the stomach through the relaxed gastro-oesophageal/cardiac sphincter.

The four stages of swallowing can only be adequately assessed by use of videofluroscopy. A limited amount of information can be gathered during the oral preparatory stage by observation and an external observer can also see whether the larynx elevates during stage 3. Videofluroscopy is the only way to obtain the necessary details of all four phases. This examination will normally involve swallowing different consistencies of food mixed with barium contrast material and following all phases of swallowing on screen. Video recording will allow later, more detailed analysis of the quite rapid automatic swallowing phase. This examination is normally carried out in conjunction with a radiologist and speech and language therapist with experience in dysphagia management. All rehabilitation units should have access to this facility.

Management

The management of eating and swallowing problems will clearly depend on the underlying cause or causes. Some

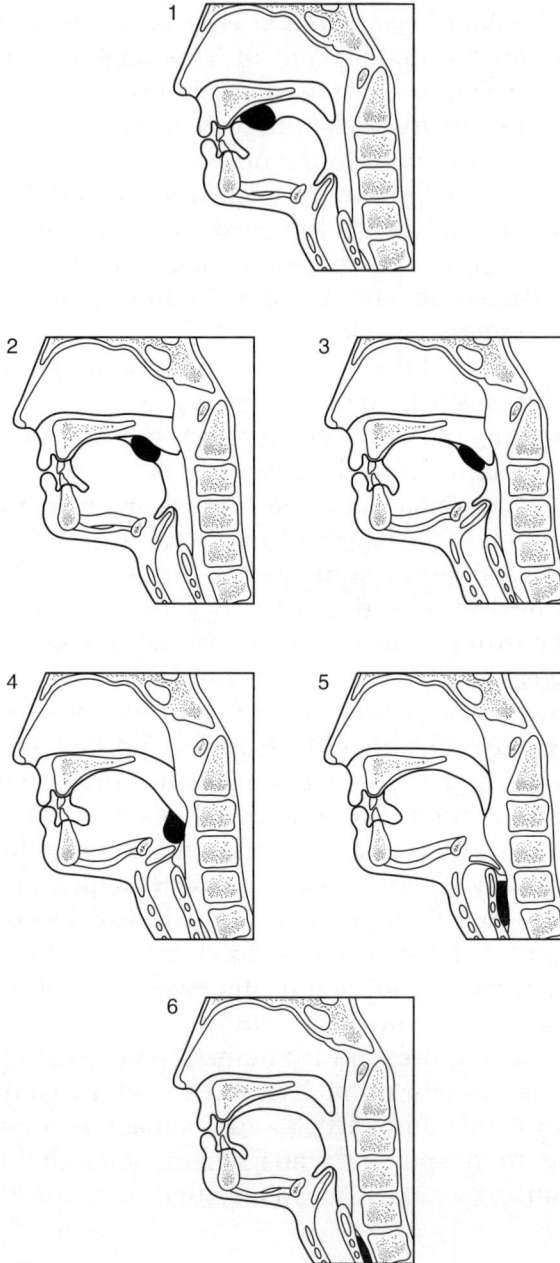

Fig. 9.1 The four stages of swallowing: (1) oral preparatory stage, (2 & 3) oral stage, (4 & 5) pharyngeal stage, (6) oesophageal stage.

obvious treatment strategies will be apparent from the assessment process outlined in the previous section. If problems of behaviour or mood, difficulties in seating or posture or with the main carer can be relieved then resulting eating and swallowing disorders should also improve.

However, if the problem lies with one of the four stages of the swallowing mechanism then a number of strategies are possible.

Modifying oral diet

A swallowing assessment, particularly videofluroscopy, will have enabled an assessment to be made of the food consistency that is best tolerated. It is often the case that thin fluids, such as soup, or crumbling food, such as biscuits, are best avoided. Usually smooth semi-solids are best, which in turn often requires thickened fluids or puréed or soft diet. At this point the advice from a dietician becomes essential. Compliance can be a problem, as such diets can be bland and strongly disliked by the individual. It is worth remembering that in the post-acute recovery phase calorific requirements are increased and sometimes up to 3000–4000 kilocalories a day are required. Increased calorie requirements are also found in some neurological conditions, particularly Huntington's chorea, and thus weight loss may not be due to a swallowing problem but simply due to an inadequate calorific intake.

The videofluroscopy may have indicated other compensatory strategies. Some guidelines that can be followed would include:

- posture—occasionally variations in head or neck posture can actually alleviate a swallowing disorder
- learning to relax and not to talk during eating can be helpful
- it is often useful to develop a feeding regime that involves small amounts of food in the mouth at one time with a quite clear deliberate chewing phase leading to a purposeful swallow
- generally several small meals a day are preferable to two or three big meals both from the point of view of swallowing and to eliminate problems with fatigue.

There is some evidence that exercises can improve oral motor control and strength and range of movement and bolus control manipulation. There are some specific techniques for a delayed swallowing reflex in which the reflex is triggered too late to prevent some aspiration. In such cases stroking of the faucial arches with a cold laryngeal mirror prior to eating seems to trigger reflex more effectively, at least in the short term. Occasionally sucking on ice can also have a similar effect.

Artificial feeding

A final resort applies to people who cannot coordinate or initiate swallowing, whose intake is too slow to be practical or for those people in whom there is a risk of aspiration of food into the larynx. For these individuals there is no safe choice but the initiation of artificial feeding. Occasionally, artificial feeding can be combined with oral intake, particularly in those who are slow as opposed to unsafe. In the short term and post-acute situation nasogastric feeding is possible. However, this does not remove the risk of aspiration and for more than a few days becomes uncomfortable and painful for the individual with some risk of ulceration. If artificial feeding is required for more than a few days then it is now standard practice to insert a percutaneous endoscopic gastrostomy (PEG) feeding tube. This is a simple procedure requiring a local anaesthetic and short-term intravenous sedation. The success rate of PEG is very high and with a very low complication rate of around 1 per cent. PEG feeding does not entirely eliminate the risk of aspiration from inhaled saliva but the risk is certainly much reduced. Obviously there are psychological problems following the removal of the normal pleasurable sensation of eating and there may be major ethical problems in people with degenerative neurological conditions, such as motor neuron disease, regarding the merits of PEG feeding. However, overall PEG feeding has made the long-term management of severe swallowing difficulties much easier and much safer.

Conclusions

Eating and swallowing disorders are common and can lead to major complications if unrecognized or untreated. Assessment is usually straightforward and videofluroscopy is a well tolerated procedure. Often straightforward advice and simple compensatory strategies are sufficient to alleviate the problem. In a small number of people artificial feeding is required. The advent of PEG tubes has simplified this problem. Overall a rehabilitation team, especially regional centres, should clearly have access to a speech and language therapist with expertise in dysphagia. The cooperation of the local radiology department and a dietician is also essential. Appropriate strategies can, of course, involve the whole rehabilitation team, particularly nursing staff, as well as the family and carers. It is essential for everyone involved with the individual to know and understand the feeding regime. The author well remembers an individual with severe aspirational problems who despite artificial feeding still had recurrent chest infections. It was only after some time that it was discovered that a close relative was regularly bringing in Mars bars which were eaten and then aspirated by the head injured individual. Communication, as always, is an essential pre-requisite for a safe feeding regime.

Further reading

Dobkin, B. H. (1996). *Neurological rehabilitation*, pp.148, 161. Davis, Philadelphia.

Fuller, D. P., Pugh, D. B., and Landau, W. M. (1994). Management of communication and swallowing disorders. In: Illis, L. S. (ed.) *Neurological rehabilitation*, pp.409–27. Blackwell Scientific, Oxford.

Groher, M. E. (1992). *Dysphagia—diagnosis and management*. Butterworth-Heinemann, London.

Lazar, R. B. and Rubkin, S. M. (1994). Speech therapy and communication disorders in neurological rehabilitation. In: Good, D. C. and Couch, J. R. (ed.) *Handbook of neurorehabilitation*, pp.219–41. Marcel Dekker, New York.

10

Communication

Despite its importance, communication is usually not well covered during basic medical training. It encompasses speech, non-verbal communication, special senses (the ability to hear and to see) and is reliant on normal cognitive function. It is often impaired in both congenital and acquired brain disorders, but more mundane problems can result in their significant deficit. While speech and language therapists have a major role to play in the assessment of communication and in the treatment of its disorders, it falls upon the whole rehabilitation team to be skilled in its appreciation and management. People with communication disorders often feel that it is the world at large that has the problem and the subsequent disability is frequently poorly appreciated. As a result, a great deal of anger can be generated by professionals unable to understand the impaired individual. Those with pure motor speech deficits on the other hand, usually understand that they have a problem and are immensely frustrated by it.

Who should be referred for communication assessment?

It is important that patients with impaired communication have access to a speech and language therapist. Assessment may take quite a long time, even in skilled hands, and other professionals simply do not have the time or the expertise to make a thorough appreciation of the problems. Care should be given to ensuring that at the time of referral, the patient can actually cope with and understand the assessment process. Speech and language therapists are concerned with all aspects of communication in terms of assessments of therapy for speech and language, improving communication skills in general, even in areas of non-verbal communication, and can pass on that advice to the rest of the rehabilitation team. It is very important that a consistent approach is given to patients by all members of the treating staff to produce the appropriate response or reply in order to reduce the frustration to a minimum.

Speech and language disorders

Four main groups of speech and language disorders exist in disabled people, which are:
- disorders of speech
- disorders of language
- disorders of fluency
- disorders of voice.

Disorders of speech

Speech or articulation disorders result in slurring. This is different from language which refers to vocabulary and to grammar, as well as to reading and writing. Articulation depends on a normal musculature and there may be many causes for impairment. Damage to the tongue, the lips, the palate, the vocal cords, or the lungs, may affect both the tone and quality. The classical articulation disorder is seen in the cleft palate, which produces a hypernasal sound. Damage to articulation can occur in the response to resuscitation following a stroke or traumatic brain injury. Loss of neuromuscular control of the structures involved in articulation due to a central or peripheral nerve lesion, results in a change of tone, coordination, or precision, resulting in *dysarthric speech*. Careful analysis of the disorder can indicate the level of the neurological lesion, as the varying characteristics change according to the site of the lesion. *Anarthria* is used to describe complete loss of speech due to impairment of neuromuscular control.

Disorders of language

Language is characterized by four elements, which are expression, comprehension, reading, and writing. The most common cause of a dysphasia is a stroke affecting the dominant hemisphere in the parietal and temporal areas. Reading and writing may also be affected, but where receptive lesions are noted, this tends to suggest a more extensive lesion. Global dysphasia suggests impairment of all aspects of language and the patient may only be able to make unintelligible grunting sounds.

Disorders of fluency

Stammering or stuttering results from hesitations and blocking of speech and tends to be less common in adults. Chronic neurological disease (spinal cord injury and multiple sclerosis in particular) can produce intercostal and diaphragmatic muscle weakness, which reduces breath control and thus fluency.

Disorders of voice

Dysphonia may be organic or psychological. Polyps, nodules, and oedema of the vocal cords cause abnormal stresses and tensions and are commonly found in singers. Although speech is usually intelligible, it is quite embarrassing for people, as it may affect the ability of people to regain work. Typical examples are from local laryngeal damage in surgery.

Commonly associated diseases

Stroke

About 15 per cent of stroke sufferers will have a significant dysphasia. Posterior inferior lesions of the temporal lobe

affect comprehension, whereas posterior superior lesions
and frontal lobe lesions affect motor functions and cause an
expressive dysphasia. The patient should be assessed as
early as possible after the stroke in order to set up a communication system with staff, family, etc. Inability to communicate is one of the most distressing features of stroke.
It is very important to ascertain how much retained ability
there is and how much reading and writing and comprehension are affected. Language disorders usually recover
only quite slowly and it may be many months or even years
before one can rule out any further improvement. The
patient should be encouraged to practice as much as he or
she is able along the guidelines set out by the speech and
language therapist and rehabilitation team.

Many patients suffer a dysarthria for a short period after
stroke and, for the most part, this recovers well. This is
typical in non-dominant parietal lobe lesions where there
may also be a loss of non-verbal communication. Severe
disability can result from an inability to appreciate the
intonation of words and the change in fluency.

Traumatic brain injury

It is difficult to know how many people are affected by
communication disorders in traumatic brain injury. There
is a high incidence of both dysphasia and articulation
problems, but speech often returns quite quickly in contrast
to stroke patients. The main difficulties in traumatic brain
injury lie in non-verbal communication and cognitive
deficits, which impair communication greatly. The speech
and language therapist works with the rest of the
rehabilitation team to find a consistent way in which to
approach and communicate with the disabled individual.
Close cooperation with clinical psychologists is vital.

Multiple sclerosis

Multiple sclerosis classically produces a spastic dysarthria
in the later stages of the disease. If the patient is ataxic, an
ataxic dysarthria can also occur. This can sometimes be
severe enough to impair communication and may also be

associated with difficulties around the tongue and mouth. As a result, feeding difficulties may occur.

Other chronic neurological diseases

The classic diseases to affect speech are Parkinson's disease, motor neuron disease, and myasthenia gravis. They all produce dysarthrias and dysphonias, and patients with Parkinson's disease classically get quieter as the disease progresses. The on–off periods of disease control affect speech greatly and very often one can judge the symptom control on speech alone. Nearly all patients with motor neuron disease will eventually become dysarthric and a significant number anarthric.

Cerebral palsy

Cerebral palsy produces many forms of dysarthria and dysphonia, but language disorders are less common and are usually associated with learning disabilities. Speech and language therapy is now available in mainstream schools and it is hoped that all these children will be able to have a formal assessment. Many at present are not comprehensively assessed until they are adults and very often they have missed out on necessary communication aids. Signing systems such as hand signs, Makaton, or Bliss signs can improve communication and the input of a speech and language therapist is very important here. Communication is a major feature of children's assessment, as they leave paediatric care, in order to allow them to compete as well as possible for places at college and in occupational activities.

Communication aids

Communication aids can be useful substitutes for speech. Where there is a severe dysarthria which makes speech unintelligible, or where there is an expressive dysphasia, the use of a simple communication aid can transform the person's life. They tend to be less helpful where there is a receptive disorder and users require considerable motivation, which rules out their use in some people with cognitive or learning difficulties.

Aids can be grouped into three types:

1. Direct/select:This is a technique which uses part of a body to indicate a symbol. An example of this is the Canon communication aid, which is a small hand-held method of typing words for communication. The moderately intelligent dysarthric or dysphasic person may prefer to use a word board which can point to the letters. Some people become very adept at writing out words.

2. Scanning: This method is chosen for people with very severe physical disabilities and a series of options comes up on a screen. The user can then point or signal the correct choice through scanning the screen.

3. Encoding: This may be used by cognitively intact people, who wish to use a relatively large vocabulary. Even though it may be limited shortly after the stroke, encoding methods are ambitious. These are probably the least commonly prescribed, but can be combined with both direct selection scanning and with environmental control equipment.

Follow-up of patients

While dysphasic patients may take some time to improve, it is essential that they are followed up. Users of communication aids must be checked to make certain that they are using them correctly. Very often, patients give up communication aids because they can use non-verbal communication very well and can communicate with their friends and family. In this instance, the aid should be returned to the speech and language therapy department. More extensive communication aids can be obtained from regional centres, such as the Access to Communication Technology. In all instances however, patients can be helped by making sure that the aid is valuable to them in their everyday lives and that they do not simply look upon it as purely for therapy.

Conclusions

The speech and language therapist has a major role within the rehabilitation team in the control of communication disorders and dysphagia. Junior doctors would benefit from an attachment to a speech and language therapist to see exactly how this role is carried out.

Further reading

Glennen, S. (1992). Augmentative and alternative communication. In: Church, G. and Glennen, S. (ed.). T*he handbook of assistive technology*, pp.93–122. Chapman and Hall, London.
Yorkston, K. M. (1992). *Augmentative communication in the medical setting*. Communication Skill Builders, Arizona.

11

....

Other physical problems

There are many physically disabling conditions, which do not conveniently fit into either diagnosis- or impairment-based classifications. This chapter will include some of them and, in particular, will address the following headings: pressure sores; contractures; pain within the context of physical disability; and the chronic fatigue syndrome (meningo-encephalitis or ME syndrome), including fibromyalgia.

Impairments of special senses will, however, not be covered, as they fall outside the authors' expertise, but the importance and impact of visual and hearing impairments is appreciated, particularly when associated with other physical disabilities. The reader should therefore seek a more authoritative text elsewhere, if further reading is required.

Pressure sores

Pressure sores are areas of erythema under the skin and may progress to ulceration and subcutaneous tissue necrosis as a result of ischaemia due to unrelieved pressure. Not only do they cause significant mortality and morbidity in themselves, but are a cause of disability and much human misery and have until recently been greatly over-looked. Although 95 per cent are totally preventable, they unfortunately still readily occur. The cost to the Health Service is immense and 3 to 11 per cent of all patients admitted to hospital develop a pressure sore. The secret of successful clinical management lies in knowing how to prevent sores developing. They are caused by ischaemia and by damage to subcutaneous blood vessels. In healthy people, the skin is very resilient, but, when one becomes ill, persistent erythema, indicative of damage, can develop within a few hours. In addition, the skin of immobile people often sticks to bed sheets and movements therefore set up friction forces, which cause injury to blood vessels in the skin, which in turn results in ischaemia, cell necrosis, and superficial ulceration. Deeper structures may be affected by shear forces occurring in the neighbourhood of bony prominences, which give rise to more extensive subcutaneous destruction. The necrotic tissue invariably becomes infected, causing inflammation of surrounding tissues and systemic toxicity. Maceration of the skin by sweat and urine reduces its tensile strength and the elderly are at special risk because ageing decreases the skin's tolerance to stress and increases the likelihood of break-down.

Clinical features and staging

Pressure sores are commonest over bony prominences such as the sacrum, buttocks, greater trochanters, ankles, and heels. The patient often feels unwell in the presence of deep infection, and putrefaction in extensive necrotic ulcers has a characteristic gangrenous odour. The clinical staging of pressure sores is shown in Table 11.1.

Despite the publicity and activity surrounding pressure sore prevention and management, prevention is still often accorded a low priority among clinicians. Most Trusts now have tissue viability specialists among the nursing staff and there is much better organization in documentation of patients at risk and in management strategies with a written policy for tissue viability and for the prevention of pressure sores.

Table 11.1 Clinical staging of pressures sores

Stage	Description	Healing
1	Discoloration of intact skin including non-blanchable erythema or loss of epidermis	Starts at surface and progresses inwards. Heals within weeks
2	Partial skin loss involving epidermis and dermis.	Starts at surface and progresses inwards. Heals within weeks
3	Full thickness skin loss extending to subcutaneous tissues	Starts deep and causes skin necrosis from below. Takes months to heal.
4	Full thickness skin loss with extensive destruction involving muscle and bone and other deep structures with tissue necrosis.	Starts deep and causes skin necrosis from below. Takes months to heal.

Who is at risk?

Table 11.2 outlines the risk factors associated with pressure sores. Immobility and severe physical disease are the commonest but all in-patients are at risk and not just those with chronic disabling disease. Sores are more commonly found in disabled people but systemic factors are associated with more severe grades. Patients with spinal or limb deformity have abnormal loads placed upon weight-bearing areas of skin and those with neurological dysfunction are also at great risk. Similarly, patients with immobilized fractured limbs and those with orthoses experience local pressure from the appliances. Particular care is required in the elderly, the obese, the cachectic, and those with impaired consciousness or physical disabilities, particularly from neurological causes. Elderly patients are at higher risk when they are admitted to hospital and in one study, 66 per cent of patients developed a pressure sore after a femoral fracture with 83 per cent of these occurring within five days of admission.

Table 11.2 Risk factors associated with pressure sores

Immobility	Neurological disease, especially tetra/paraplegia
	Obesity
	Coma/confusion
Sensory loss	Severe physical disease
	Weight loss
	Low albumin
	Low vitamin C
Deformity	Producing abnormal loads
	Redundancy
	Fractures
	Faecal and urinary incontinence

Scores have been developed to identify patients at risk and the Norton and Waterlow scores are the best known and have been validated. The former unfortunately does not take nutritional status into account which is obviously of importance. The Waterlow scale is given in figure 11.1.

Prevention

Pressure sores do not occur in situations where doctors, nurses, and therapists have an interest in pressure sore prevention. Good communication between members of the team and regular inspections of pressure areas in *all* patients in a ward is necessary. These inspections should be more frequent in patients who are at risk or in the high-risk category. Just because a patient is on an anti-pressure sore mattress or seating does not obviate the need for frequent turning. This is the essential mechanism of pressure sore prevention.

At-risk patients

In addition to frequent turning and inspection of at-risk patients, education is most important. Turning should be every two hours during the day and three hours at night,

Build/weight for height

	*
Average	0
Above average	1
Obese	2
Below average	3

Continence

	*
Complete	0
Catheterised	1
Occassion incont.	
Cath/incontinenet of faeces	2
Doubly incont.	3

Skin type visual risk areas

	*
Healthy	0
Tissue paper	1
Dry	1
Oedematours	1
Clammy (temp ↑)	1
Discoloured	2
Broken/spot	3

Mobility

	*
Fully	0
Restless/fidgety	1
Apathetic	2
Restricted	3
Inert/traction	4
Chairbound	5

Sex Age

	*
Male	1
Female	2
14–49	1
50–64	2
65–74	3
75–80	4
80+	5

Appetite

	*
Average	0
Poor	1
N.G. tube/	
Fluids only	2
NBM/anorexia	3

Special risks

Tissue malnutrition

	*
e.g. Terminal cachexia	8
Cardiac failure	5
peripheral vascular disease	5
Anaemia	2
Smoking	1

Neurological deficit

	*
e.g.: Diabetes, M.S., CVA, Motor/sensory, Paraplegia	4–6

Major surgery/trauma

	*
Orthopeadic below waist, spinal	5
on table > 2 hours	5

Medication

	*
Steroids, cytotoxics, High dose anti-inflammatory	4

Score	10+ At risk	15+ High risk	70+ Very high risk

Fig. 11.1 Waterlow pressure sore prevention/treatment policy. Ring scores in table, add total. Several scores per category can be used.

although once per night tends to be sufficient in many younger patients with a spinal injury. A designated key worker should be involved with every patient to ensure that pressure sores do not occur. There should be a well established system for provision and replacing of mattresses and beds and wheelchairs should be correctly fitted to prevent sores. Foam cushions 3 in thick are suitable for most patients, together with instructions to relieve pressure areas regularly. Those at highest risk may need special seating such as gel or air cell cushions, and specialized assessment should be obtained from the district wheelchair service.

Management

If pressure sores develop, treatment comprises general supportive measures, topical and systemic therapy and, for some patients, surgery. The principles of treatment are much the same for all sores, whether they occur on the trunk or on the limbs. Factors delaying healing should be addressed, which may include poor nutritional state, anaemia etc.

Relief of pressure is the most important factor, and incontinence of faeces and urine should be controlled. It is useful to ensure that faecal loading and constipation do not exist and, if haematinics are ineffective at maintaining a haemoglobin above 10 g dl^{-1}, transfusion should be considered. A good diet containing protein and vitamin C is essential.

The principle of treatment is to remove pressure by keeping the patient off the affected part as much as possible. Topical treatments are available and different formulae have different functions:

1. Semi-permeable films to cover ulcers and sooth the skin.
2. Antiseptic agents to reduce infection.
3. Dressings to absorb exudate: alginate dressings, hydrocolloid, and hydrogel systems.
4. Agents to remove slough, which include enzymes as well as hydrocolloid and hydrogel systems.
5. Agents to promote granulation tissue.

Systemic therapy

Antibiotics are unnecessary unless infection is caused by invasion of deep structures by the sore. Bony infection requires long courses of effective antibiotics, and both anti-staphylococcal and anti-anaerobic organism agents are required.

Surgery

The indications for surgery are to debride necrotic material and to cover a clean ulcer with good granulation tissue. It is sometimes possible to perform a primary repair, but surgery should be seen as an adjunct to conservative therapy rather than its substitute. Medical staff should not be afraid to debride an ulcer on the ward, particularly in insensate patients, as this will speed up the healing process. Formal plastic and reconstructive surgery to provide skin and muscle flaps is often required in weight-bearing areas around the buttock and sacrum and over the trochanters, as a graft will often not survive the stresses and strains.

Conclusion

Most pressure sores are preventable and if they do develop, are very costly to treat. A high level of awareness among all staff and carers is required and guidelines to optimal prevention and care must be strictly followed by all staff.

Contractures

Tendon and joint contracture occurs in prolonged immobility, due to either neurological or musculoskeletal pathology. The lesion starts with muscle and tendon shortening or joint capsule restriction, thereby leading to fibrosis and loss of range of movement across articulations and limbs. The process may start as a result of pain in a limb, joint disease, spasticity, or simple poor positioning. The resultant restriction of limb movement leads to loss of function, and thus loss of dexterity, mobility, etc. As a result, much time must be spent in stretching the limbs in order to reverse the process and contractures lead to severe problems with perineal hygiene with pain, inability to place the foot flat on the ground, loss of dexterity, and, notably, poor self-esteem and mood changes.

Treatment is difficult and is often painful, but where contractures are established, serial splinting, using a plaster of Paris cast should be attempted. The limb is stretched and the plaster of Paris cast is applied. New resins have allowed rapidly setting casts, which makes this process easier. The cast is left for 7 to 10 days and then removed. The limb is then stretched further and a new cast is applied. Very often, back slabs are used instead of cylindrical casts to facilitate inspection of the limb and allow physiotherapy. Where return of limb function is not possible, as in patients with severe hemiplegia or paraplegia, tenotomy or arthrotomy operations may be needed to allow tissue release and further stretching is applied.

Chronic pain

The management of chronic pain is vastly different from that of acute pain. The common conditions associated with chronic musculoskeletal pain are neck and back pain, occupational upper limb disorders, degenerative joint disease, and reflex sympathetic dystrophy (Sudek's atrophy). Analgesics do not control the situation and the ensuing disability arises from a combination of the physical disorder, anxiety, and a form of illness behaviour.

The management of chronic pain requires particular skills in knowledge of the underlying condition and in communicating with patients and their families. Pain relief clinics have been established throughout the country and have to a greater or lesser extent been reasonably successful. However, pain in the context of physical disability has been less well addressed and rehabilitation physicians, through their training in communicating with patients and in their interactions with members of a multidisciplinary team, can make a significant contribution to this issue. Chronic symptoms due to mechanical or degenerative disease require a coping strategy and, when medical treatments are inappropriate or cease to be effective, follow-up is required to support the patient and family. The organization of pain relief clinics probably failed to do this adequately and some are primarily used for pain-relieving procedures rather than as a holistic approach to the patient's problems. Described below are three specific pain syndromes.

Central pain syndromes

Thalamic pain following stroke or traumatic brain injury can be very disabling and usually leads to dysaesthesia or an awareness of sensation in the affected area of the body, very often down one side. The crucial lesion is often in the spinathalamo-cortical pathway which is responsible for pain and temperature sensing, and disordered function is thought to be the cause. Pain may occur soon after the event or be delayed for many months. Patients can often experience more than one type of pain. Movement, touch, cold, especially a cold breeze, can often bring on the pain.

Various treatments have been applied, including anti-depressant medication, anti-convulsants, (in particular Carbamazepine, sodium valproate, and Gabapentin) muscle relaxants and effusions, and even Chlorpromazine. No one particular treatment has been validated and none are routinely successful.

Reflex neurovascular dystrophy/reflex sympathetic dystrophy/Sudek's atrophy

This is a group of disorders in which an injury or insult proximally can lead to pain distally in the limb. This pain is continuous in nature and is accompanied by hyperalgesia and allodynia. Local abnormal sympathetic activity is observed, with changes in temperature and colour of the limb and abnormal sweating. The affected part becomes cold and pale and muscles become wasted. Contractures and osteopenia appear, giving the name of Sudek's atrophy, and sympathetic blockade is the treatment of choice. This

should be combined with active exercise and physiotherapy and other measures of chronic pain relief, such as
anti-depressant medication.

Management of pain

The patient should be thoroughly assessed in order to
devise a treatment plan in which the participation of the
patient and carer is essential. Where patients have been
complaining of pain for years from degenerative disease,
further medical intervention may be inappropriate and this
should be clearly communicated. In this context, community rehabilitation teams with participation from social
workers and non-health-related professionals should be
to the fore of a management strategy. However, painful
exacerbations need to be treated with effective medication
and mild, but active, exercise. Patients should be responsible for their own management and should seek medical
assistance only when initial measures have failed. Successful management is critically dependent on finding a
regimen of treatment which will help the patient. A
combined approach of physical exercise, medication and
other therapies is required for most patients.

Physical treatments and exercise

Prolonged physiotherapy for people with chronic pain
increases dependence on health professionals and patients
should be taught an exercise programme that encompasses
general exercise to improve fitness, specific exercises to
protect the affected part of the body, and information on
how to deal with painful exacerbations. Manipulation and
mobilization may be useful for this and for reducing muscle
spasm and pain in acute situations, but there is no evidence
that they or other treatments alter the natural history of
chronic pain.

Medication

Centrally acting analgesics are obviously useful, but can
cause sedation and constipation. Starting off with simple
medication and increasing the dose and the potency of
these opioid analgesics can be effective, but again, patients

with chronic pain due to a wide variety of causes will often get a ceiling effect. Narcotic analgesics suppress natural endorphine production and can be quite dependent. They thus have real place in the management of chronic pain.

Tricyclic anti-depressants have been shown to be of most use in treating anxiety and depression in chronic pain and probably have a synergistic action with analgesics. They should be used for periods of 3 to 6 months as shorter periods of time are often ineffective. Both tricyclic anti-depressants and selective serotonin re-uptake inhibitors (SSRIs) have an equal impact on pain relief, although some examples in these groups have a better action than others. Paroxetine tends to be more helpful in this situation than Fluoxetine as it has a more sedative action. Similarly, both Amitriptyline and Dothiepin are useful in inducing sleep when taken at night, and thus a reasonable period of rest allows the patient to be more resilient to cope with the following day.

Specific injections
Local injections of corticosteroids into joints can be helpful in reducing active synovitis, even in the absence of overt inflammation. Local nerve blocks relieve pain in a multitude of conditions ranging from soft tissue problems to intractable pain from osteoarthritis. Subscapular nerve blocks are easy to do and are very effective in intractable shoulder pain. Regional sympathetic blockage is useful in many conditions, ranging from inflammatory joint disease to osteoarthritis and to reflex neurovascular dystrophy. Although the effects are sometimes short-lived, the procedure is relatively straightforward. Even more simple, are Guanethedine blockade of distal limbs, using 20 mg of Guanethidine intravenously in a cuffed limb.

Epidural injections are useful for acute and acute intermittent pain, but long-term relief has not been demonstrated in chronic settings. They allow sufficient pain relief, using a mixture of corticosteroid and long-acting local anaesthetic such as Bupivacaine and allow the patient to exercise and mobilize the spine thereafter.

Facet joint injection is useful in the facet joint syndrome and in lumbar spondylosis, although the evidence does not tend to support this in patient populations. It is probably of value in very specific patients, in whom there is referred pain and localized tenderness over the joint in question. Joints should thus be tender and injections are invariably more effective when one single joint is at fault. Local tenderness and pain on extension and rotation of the spine are key diagnostic factors and the effect of injections, which should be done under the image intensifier to ensure accuracy, can allow relief of pain for several weeks if not months.

Muscle relaxants
These probably have little role in the treatment of chronic pain. Baclofen and Dantrolene sodium are sometimes used for their anti-spastic qualities, but again, since the spasm is purely pain-induced, they are unlikely to be of real benefit in either the short or long term. Additionally, they cause considerable side effects and should probably not be used. Benzodiazepines are good muscle relaxants, but are significantly addictive and produce side effects on withdrawal. Their long-term use is not recommended.

Other treatments
Treatment with transcutaneous nerve stimulation (TNS) or acupuncture is effective in reducing the amount of pain that the patient will experience. They can also be used in combination with other treatments and require suitable education to ensure their efficacy. TNS is found in most physiotherapy departments and acupuncture should be carried out by trained personnel.

   Corsets and braces can be helpful for acute exacerbations, but lead to disuse atrophy of muscles when used long term. They should thus be avoided and the muscles should be built up with remedial exercise.

Cognitive behavioural therapy
This involves developing certain behavioural characteristics in respect of trying to normalize activities in chronic pain. One therefore encourages the patient to attempt certain key tasks every day and follows this up with rest and evaluation of the pain level. It has had an effect in many

patients and the aim is to develop a coping strategy for participation in day-to-day activities. Time is of the essence here and consistency of approach results in a better response.

Chronic fatigue syndrome/fibromyalgia

This unknown group of disorders has become quite topical in the media over recent years, but formal studies have failed to show the underlying pathology. There is no doubt that it produces genuine symptom complexes of widespread musculoskeletal pain, severe fatiguability, and functional disturbance at many levels. There is hyperalgesia, tenderness at specific sites, and marked fatigue. Table 11.3 shows the possible mechanism for this syndrome. The ME syndrome of fibromyalgia has been categorized together under Chronic Fatigue Syndrome, but it is not known whether they are truly related. The wide variation of symptoms and signs suggests that it is all one and the same thing. Although fibromyalgia has been recognized for many years as a distinct entity, the ME syndrome is relatively new and some say that it has been 'forced on' the medical professional by interested groups. However, the symptoms and disability caused by this condition are real, and are not fabricated or imagined (Table 11.4). The cause of the disability is functional rather than pathological and the tenderness and associated sleep disturbance are characteristic. This can be reproduced by selective deprivation of non-REM sleep and appears to be universally present in these patients.

Fibromyalgia is classified as primary and secondary, when underlying pathology can be identified, such as osteoarthritis. Patients are often anxious or depressed and women are more commonly affected than men. It is often thought to be a condition of higher social classes, but there is no evidence for this. Patients are often anxious about other underlying diseases such as cancer or multiple sclerosis and investigation often includes an MR scan for the chronic fatigue syndrome to rule out MS. Similarly, in true fibromyalgia, inflammatory joint disease must be ruled

Table 11.3 Diagnostic terms in fibromyalgia

Principal presenting symptom	Diagnostic label
Locomotor pain	Fibrositis, pain amplification syndrome, fibromyalgia
Fatigue	ME syndrome, chronic fatigue syndrome
Headache	Tension headache
Abdominal pain, bowel disturbance	Irritable bowel syndrome

Table 11.4 Some common symptoms of fibromyalgia

Symptom	Description
Pain	Predominantly neck and back aggravated by stress and by cold. Generalized morning stiffness following activity, generalized pain, poor response to analgesics
Fatiguability	Follows even minimal exertion and may be severe
Other	Subjective limb swelling, paraesthesiae, dysaesthesia of hands and feet, poor sleep, poor concentration, low mood, irritability, weakness, headache, often occipital or bifrontal, diffuse abdominal pain, variable bowel habit, urgency of micturition

out, along with hypothyroidism, hyperparathyroidism, osteomalacia, inflammatory myopathy, and systemic lupus erythematosus.

Management

The initial and perhaps the most important aspect of management is to reassure the patient that they have a genuine condition, and it is not due to their imagination. Nor are they attempting to deceive either the professionals or their families. There is often a considerable element of anxiety among both patients and their families and an over-concerned partner can often generate the problems.

Management is through a combination of anti-depressant medication with either tricyclics or selective Serotonin re-uptake inhibitors. A programme of gentle exercise can often be valuable as long as the fatigue is able to cope with this. Cognitive behavioural programmes are more frequently instituted and good close working between psychiatrists, psychologists, rheumatologists, and rehabilitationists is becoming more valuable. The basis of these programmes is to get patients to accept responsibility for their pain and their disability. The aim is to increase the patient's belief in his/her own ability to control pain and to improve energy levels. This is done by a combination of physical relaxation, stress management, and pacing of activities. Even though the pain may still cause problems, the patient eventually becomes more able to increase their social, leisure, and occupational activities. These programmes are mapped out for the individual and included in this are rest periods interspersed with increasing activities.

Conclusion

The prognosis in chronic fatigue syndrome and fibromyalgia is not particularly good. Self-help groups have been set up and there is a concern that, while patients themselves may be helped to understand their problems, the group per-petuates the sick role rather than benefits of rehabilitation.

Chronic fatigue states should be managed by people who are interested in the subject and who can reassure the patient of the genuineness of their complaint. As with so many facets of medicine, rehabilitation expertise is re-quired, and each health district should identify an appro-priate person to take on some of the load.

Further reading

The fibromyalgia syndrome. *Rheumatic Disease Clinics of North America*, (1989), **15**, (1), 1–191.

Butler, R. C. and Dayson, M. I. V. (ed.) (1985–95). *Collected Reports on the Rheumatic Diseases*, pp.83–86 and pp.132–137. Arthritis and Rheumatism, Chesterfield.

12

Technical aids and assistive technology

Technical aids

Technical aids cover all equipment for disabled people, whether for use in the home, at work, or in the community at large. They range from simple devices in the kitchen or bathroom, to hoists, stair-lifts, and any item which may improve the standard of living for a disabled person. Some are personally used by the disabled person, whereas others are designed to be operated by carers. (The maxim that the more simple the device, the more effective it is, is very true and this is typified by armchairs with elevating seats, which assist disabled people with limited hip and knee movement to rise from the chair.) In addition, this equipment is often very useful, not only for the disabled person, but for the rest of the household as well.

Occupational therapists have particular skills in assessing and recommending such pieces of equipment and many large towns and cities have disabled living centres, where a range of equipment can be viewed and inspected. The Disabled Living Foundation has a large database of information and a list of disabled living centres. Care equipment helps disabled people, but is designed to protect the carers from injury. Hoists and items to help with transfers, for instance, will protect carers from back pain and it is important that safety, as well as improvement in function, are features with which one would recommend an aid.

Assistive technology encompasses the whole array of technical equipment which reduces handicap and which allow disabled people greater independence in their lives. It covers simple technical aids, as well as electronic devices and devices which might be actually fitted to the patient and which he or she may operate within their homes or outdoors. This book could not possibly hope to cover the vast array of equipment, and the aim, therefore, is to give the reader an impression of the areas in which help may be most available, with the suggested reading at the end of this chapter allowing more specific references.

The value of professionals trained in rehabilitation is that they will have a good knowledge, not only of what is available to help disabled people, but will think pro-actively about the difficulties that may be alleviated with the use of equipment. Very often, patients are simply never given the opportunity to be helped in this way because their attending professionals just never think about this aspect of rehabilitation. This chapter will therefore look particularly at wheelchairs, special seating, orthoses, prostheses, environmental controls, and driving. Communi-cation aids are very important areas of assistive technology and are very often linked in with environmental controls. They have, however, been included in the chapter on com-munication (Chapter10).

Wheelchairs

Wheelchairs can be obtained either through the National Health Service or can be bought privately. Their provision was transferred from the Department of Health to the Dis-ablement Services Authority in 1987 following the McColl report which was published in 1986. They became part of the National Health Service provision in 1991 on the Dis-ablement Services Authority's integration into the Health Service. One of the major changes has been the development of the Wheelchair Services at local district level. Each is supported by trained therapists, usually occupational therapists, and the organization includes both rehabilitation engineers and administrative and clerical staff, who keep account of the service activities and contracts. Consultants in rehabilitation medicine usually have considerable involvement with these services and the whole principle of the McColl report was that a wheelchair service should be integrated with rehabilitation services. Disabled people have many needs, of which one is mobility. Their mobility may require, or be enhanced by, a wheelchair and this provision is part of the overall rehabilitation aim for that particular patient. In this context, disabled people have identified specific needs and may require more than one wheelchair—for work, at college, and at home. Services therefore have to be flexible and sensitive to these needs. The result is that each individual is assessed on his or her own merits, obviously within the constraints of some fundamental parameters. Again the range of available equipment changes in different situations. Students may be able to manage a manual wheelchair over the shorter distances in their homes, but may not be able to manage longer distances at college and therefore may require an electric powered chair.

Prescription of a wheelchair

A chair is obtained by completion of the local referral form, which is then sent to the wheelchair service following a doctor's signature. This form should be filled out as accurately as possible, as patients need the appropriate chair as much as they need accuracy from prescription for a drug. NHS Wheelchair Services only prescribe chairs to people who are likely to require them for more than six months. There are exceptions to this rule, such as for patients with rapidly progressive disorders. It is also worth noting that some patients will require to spend many hours in their wheelchair, if they are obligatory users, whereas some chairs will be used only on an intermittent basis. As the population ages, more and more chairs are prescribed to elderly people just to allow them to get down to the shops once a week for a few hours or so. The main considerations in wheelchair prescription are listed below:

1. Diagnosis
2. Frequency of the chair's use
3. Where will the chair be used?—Outdoors? Indoors? Both? Local environmental factors
4. Transfers in and out of the chair—unaided, standing, sideways, assisted by carer, transfer boards, etc. Should arm rests be removable to allow sideways transfer?
5. Transportation of chair.
6. Needs of carer
7. Seating—need for cushion, special seating or complex seating system, activities in the chair, other factors, e.g. incontinence.

The diagnosis is important to give the prescriber essential information on the usage of the chair, the need for review, and on the speed of delivery. For instance, someone with a malignancy or motor neuron disease may require a chair more urgently than an elderly person who has simply become frail. Practical considerations, such as the client's ability to transfer, have obviously to be taken into consideration. Detaching the armrests and the provision of footrests form part of this assessment and therefore information on both the client and carer is very important. Complicating factors, such as severe spasticity, may interfere with comfortable sitting and with transfers and should always be mentioned in the referral form. The height and fitness of the carer is also crucial. If it is necessary to transport the chair in a car, then the carer's ability to lift the equipment into the boot is vital. Less dependent disabled people may wish to transport their own chair, say on the roof of their vehicle, and further information is required of their skills.

Not every client requires an individual assessment for their chair. For instance, someone wishing to take Granny out occasionally does not require a complex assessment or a seating system. However, the wheelchair requires to be individually adjusted at all times on delivery. Those with complex problems do require to be seen in a wheelchair clinic and medical input into these is of great value. A wheelchair user should ideally be able to sit straight in a chair in a comfortable position. The thigh should be parallel to the ground and the footrest should allow the foot to be at a right angle to the lower leg. The armrests should be adjusted so that the forearm is again parallel to the ground and that the elbow is in line to the trunk to allow a 90° angle. The user should be able to sit within a 15° angle of upright to be comfortable in the chair.

Types of wheelchair

There are four main categories of chair, ranging from a push-chair or buggy, a manual self-propelled chair, an attendant-propelled chair, and finally a powered chair. Pushchairs and buggies are mainly for disabled children and have many similar features to those found for young able-bodied children. They require to be supportive, but easy to use and should be able to fold away. As children get older, they may require special seating (see below) and will then move on to a junior wheelchair. These have similar features to adult wheelchairs, whose main differences are those which can be propelled by the disabled individual and those who have to be pushed by an attendant.

There are now a large number of different models, which are characterized by the size of the seat and the weight of the chair. An NHS 8LJ chair is a junior version of the 8L standard 16 in seat and the 8BL is a 15 in by 16 in seat. Larger 8L chairs are available, with seat widths up to 20 in, but difficulties then arise in manoeuvring a chair around the house and getting it through doorways etc. NHS 9 series wheelchairs come in the same sizes as the 8 series, but have four small wheels and are only designed for propulsion by an attendant. The NHS has been able to provide self-propelling electric-powered chairs for indoor use only, but since 1 April 1997 it is now possible for those regular indoor-powered chair users to have uprated chairs for outside use also. Before 1997, attendant-controlled electric outdoor chairs were available from the NHS but were large, heavy, cumbersome, and were undesirable to many disabled people.

Various features can be attached to chairs to improve the user's comfort. These include trunk supports, altered armrests, tilting backrests, head supports, and adjustable footrests. More sporty wheelchairs are also now available through NHS provision, which have a greater 'street credibility' amongst the young. Obviously, the type of wheelchair should be matched to the patient's abilities to get around and the underlying condition and the age and fitness of the user will be critical within the context of the chair's use inside and outside the home. Some lighter weight wheelchairs have a rigid frame to provide stability and these of course will not fold. They can be transported by removal of their wheels, but are somewhat cumbersome for many people. Heavier wheelchairs can thus sometimes be more practical since they do fold, but it must also be remembered that electric powered chairs again do not fold. If they require to be transported, their batteries may need to be removed and this causes additional risks of damage to the batteries. Tetraplegics above the level of C5 will most probably require an electric wheelchair and control of electric chairs is usually carried out with a joystick above the control box. Less conventional means may have to be adopted, such as the use of a chin control, a blow and suck control, a head control or even a photoelectric cell. A range of wheelchairs is illustrated at Figs. 12.1–12.5.

Wheelchair services

It is valuable for all doctors to visit their local wheelchair service to find out what is available, and staff there will be more than happy to explain their role and the availability of equipment. Regional rehabilitation centres will have more specialized equipment for people with complex needs, which will usually tie up with specialized seating.

Special seating

Definition

Special seating is that component of a seating system, in either a static chair or a wheelchair, which is specifically prescribed for disabled people to accommodate or to control any postural difficulties or to manage problems that may

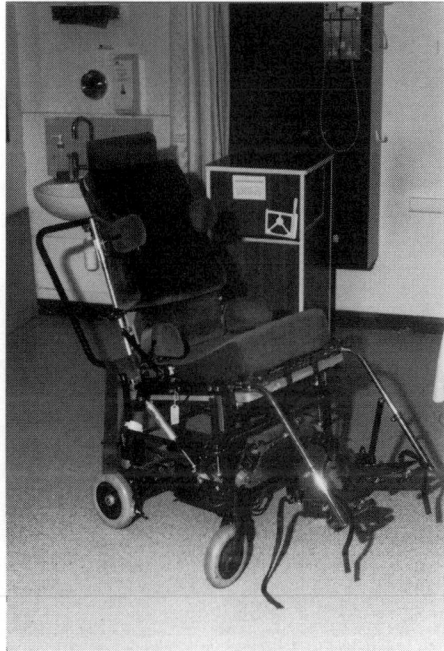

Fig. 12.1

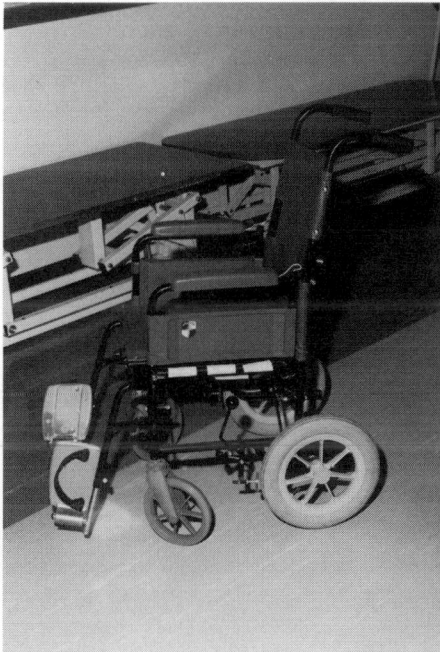

Fig. 12.2

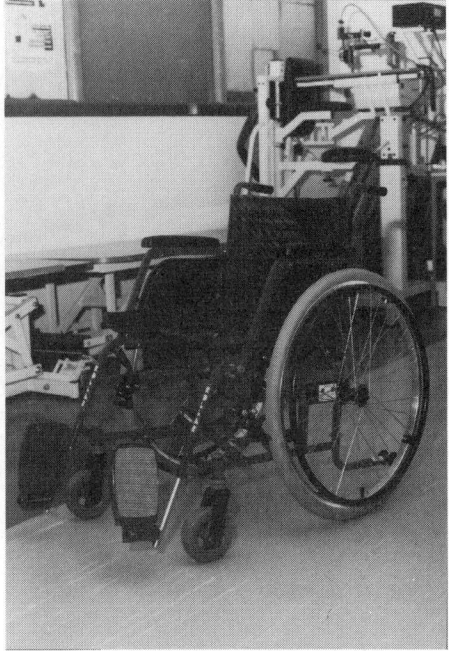

Fig. 12.3

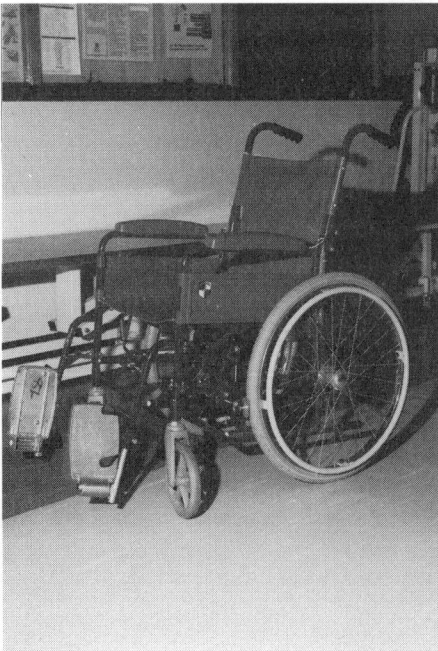

Fig. 12.4

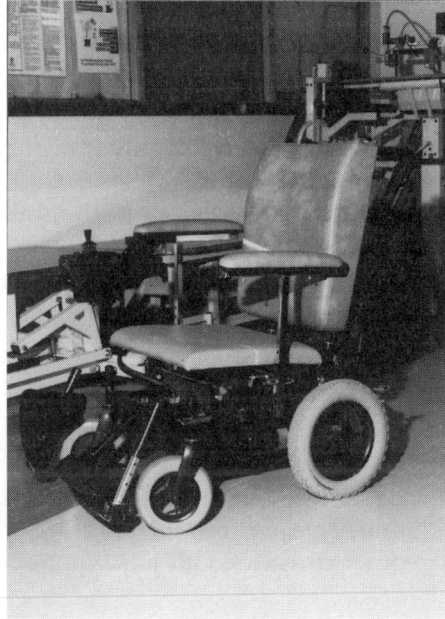

Fig. 12.5

arise from abnormal pressures due to deformity. It is primarily provided for people with moderate or severe disability, whose definition is given in Table 12.1.

Special seating is required when standard seating systems are unable to control the posture of the disabled person sufficiently. Depending on whether there is weakness and motor impairment or fixed skeletal deformity and pressure problems, special seating gives either dynamic or static support. The former allows the enhancement of functional ability, whereas static support systems maintain function and prevent deformities from worsening. In practice, most seating systems fulfil a hybrid of the two roles (Table 12.2).

The seating system depends on the severity of the disability, the abilities and requirements of the disabled person, and the ability and needs of carers and other environmental factors.

• Many seating systems are designed for children with multiple disabilities, and who therefore require seating which will cater for both physical problems and stringent safety requirements. Children with learning

Table 12.1   Definitions for special seating criteria

Mild disability
- Good head control
- Good to fair trunk control. May be unstable when sitting unsupported
- Good functional ability with minimal support when given a stable base.

Moderate disability
- By and large, good head control, but poor trunk control
- Unable to sit in a stable position without support
- Limited hand control when sitting in a stable position

Severe disability
- Poor head and trunk control
- Unable to sit without support
- Limited upper limb function
- Spinal curvature and joint contractures

difficulties often have fixed deformities as a result of poor positioning in early life and an appropriate seating system can improve their lifestyle and their self-esteem. Chronic neurological disease in adults is the commonest indication for specialized seating and spasticity and contracture formation in multiple sclerosis is a major indication in adults. As users may be spending many hours daily in their seats, great attention to detail and to comfort is mandatory. A good seating system therefore should aim to:

Table 12.2   Aims of special seating systems

Achieve stability and balance
Reduce the effort to maintain posture
Prevent or delay the onset or worsening of deformities
Optimize function
Provide comfort
Allow distribution of load to provide maximal pressure relief
Decrease cardiorespiratory burden through functional support

- Enable good positioning for comfortable sitting, for feeding, swallowing, and for communication
- Encourage bladder and bowel drainage and function
- Provide good eye contact
- Support the trunk to decrease the effort of breathing
- Provide comfort
- Be practical for carer function.

Organization of services

Special seating systems are expensive and, in the context of health care constraints, cannot be freely available, unless there is a clinical need. Simpler seating systems are prescribed by local wheelchair services, but more complex arrangements are provided by regional centres. The expertise there, from rehabilitation engineers and specialized rehabilitationists and therapists, ensures more cost-effective provision of seating systems.

Footwear and orthoses

Orthoses are devices worn outside the body which support and aid the function of that part. They and special footwear, play an important part in assisting disabled people improve personal function. It is important that all doctors and therapists acquire a basic training in orthotics at both undergraduate and postgraduate level, in order to realize their potential value. As with other technical assistance, the decision to use an orthosis should be made on team discussion. The team should include a doctor, a therapist, nursing staff, and orthotists and each orthosis should be prescribed with a specific aim. Both the orthotist and patient should have a thorough knowledge of what the orthosis is attempting to do. If the device is not worn, then the whole process fails and the technical merits of the appliance serve no useful purpose. The team should thus estimate the patient's compliance and education is an important feature.

Some orthoses are highly complex and costly and therefore close working between the doctor, therapist, and orthotist is important to make best use of scarce resources.

Orthoses are suitable for people disabled by musculo-skeletal and neurological conditions. Table 12.3 shows a simple overview of some of the commoner types. This section aims to provide the reader with a basic knowledge of the subject and the suggested further reading at the end of the chapter will give further information on more complex items.

Footwear

Foot pain is one of the commonest presentations to GPs, rheumatologists, orthopaedic surgeons, and rehabilitation physicians. It may be due to joint disease or to nerve injury from unsupported weight-bearing structures. Prevention of subtalar subluxation is important in early joint disease in order to prevent pain distally and the wearing of good footwear is a cheap and effective way to help this. Footwear has never commanded much attention from the medical profession and many doctors do not realize how prescribing comfortable shoes can transform the lives of people with painful feet. The development of depth shoes has increased the range available and there is now less need for individually made (bespoke) surgical shoes.

Insoles

Medial and longitudinal arch supports
These are used for simple flat feet, for lateral plantar nerve compression and for the prevention of subtalar valgus subluxation as commonly occurs in both rheumatoid and osteoarthritis.

Table 12.3 Types of orthoses

Footwear
- Insoles, shoe modifications, bespoke shoes

Supports
- Collars, lumbar supports/belts, epicondylitis clasps

Splints
- Static/resting (prevents movement and supports joints)
- Working/lively (helps to increase limb function)

Metatarsal domes

These devices in the shoe transfer weight away from the metatarsal heads to the metatarsal shafts and relieve the pain from metatarso-phalangeal joint disease and subluxation. A larger size of shoe may be needed to prevent callosities on the dorsum of the toes and plastazote temporary domes should first be fitted to test their efficacy.

Heel insoles

Indications are for traumatic heel and leg pain and plantar fasciitis. Occasionally a hole needs to be cut out in the insole under the tender point of the heel in order to provide more comfort, but new materials using shock-absorbing pads, can be useful in the prevention of heel pain. Sorbothane and Viscolast are two such devices.

Modified shoes

Shoe raises

These are used to correct unequal leg lengths. When leg lengths are measured and compared, it is not necessary to correct the shorter leg to equal that of the longer leg. Normally, the amount of raise needed is about half the leg length difference, so that a normal swing phase is maintained in walking. Differences of less than 1cm are probably not worth correcting in this way.

Depth shoes

These are enhanced footwear for people with deformed feet. They are lightweight with a non-slip sole and have a wide opening to allow easy fitting. Fortunately, they are fairly cheap to produce and cater for most deformities, and sufficient space is available to fit an insole. However, this should be checked first (Fig. 12.6).

Bespoke shoes

These are individually designed to fit people with difficult feet, and can fulfil a variety of functions from tough working shoes to comfortable lightweight items. They are very expensive to make and casts need to be made before

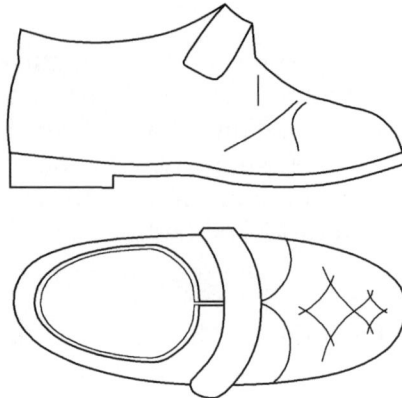

Fig. 12.6   Depth shoes.

the final shoe is manufactured. These casts should therefore be checked against the patient's feet before the manufacturing process. As a result, considerable time is consumed in making sure that they are correct, which contributes to the high cost of these shoes.

Supports

Collars
These are used to reduce pain by supporting the neck, but do not truly prevent neck movements, no matter how strong the materials used are. If effective immobilization of the head is required, skull or halo traction should be used. Collars should be comfortable, but this may be difficult to achieve in hot weather. They are useful in reduction of muscle spasm in the few days after a whiplash injury to the neck and patients with rheumatoid disease should be fitted with a collar in preparation for surgery, which will alert the anaesthetist to the risk of vertebral and spinal cord damage during intubation.

Corsets
The commonest indication for a corset is an acute lumbar disc protrusion with muscle spasm. They are usually prescribed during the mobilization phase after rest, and

are unfortunately rather uncomfortable to wear. As a result, they are often discarded, but constantly remind the wearer to protect the back, and, more importantly, they support the anterior abdominal wall. Some patients, who wear corsets for years, find themselves unable to do without them and it is inadvisable in modern practice to allow patients to rely on these supports in the long term. Polythene jackets are used with variable success for the pain of osteoporotic vertebral collapse and to prevent the effects on respiration of increasing truncal weakness as seen in muscular dystrophies etc. Again, they are often uncomfortable to wear, and patient compliance is variable.

Epicondylitis clasps

These are worn on the proximal forearm to decrease the load on the extensor and flexor muscle origins and tennis and golfer's elbow respectively. They transfer the effective origin point of the muscle to a point under the clasp through a tight grip over the muscle's belly. Since this protects the enthesis (the point of attachment of tendon to bone) at the lateral/ medial humeral epicondyle, patients are often able to work or play games while wearing the clasp.

Splints

It is possible to make splints for anything from simple thumb pain to a major brachial plexus injury. The aims and functions of splintage are described in Table 12.4 and can be generally grouped as below.

1. Resting splints. These immobilize the affected part of the limb and are often used at night to rest joints. Help may be required to apply and remove them, particularly if bilateral splints are used, and they may interfere with daily function too much to be used as anything more than night resting devices. Care thus needs to be taken before prescribing them. An example of such a device is a paddle splint incorporating the wrist and small joints of the hands for patients with active rheumatoid arthritis.

Table 12.4   Functions of a splint

Stabilize joints
Reduce pain and inflammation through immobilization
Place limb in the best functional position
Protect joints leading to confident usage
Prevent or reduce further deformity

2. Working or lively splints. These allow a limb to work in some functional way and may incorporate a moving part, either free-moving or against resistance. Stabilizing one joint may result in better functional use of the whole limb, but excessive deformity of the joint contra-indicates the wearing of a lively splint, since it may rub the underlying skin during use and impair the actual function of the device. For instance, a valgus or varus deformity of 20° in the knee is usually the maximum for which a splint can be tolerated.

3. Serial splinting. This technique is used to increase the range of movement across a joint where there is contracture of either the joint or the tendon. They are perhaps less used now than before, but still have particular indications in both musculoskeletal and neurological disease where joint and tendon abnormalities have occurred due to poor positioning of limbs or to marked spasticity. Serial splinting still has its place in rehabilitation and will reduce even very large contractures, when accompanied by active physical treatment. The limb is straightened to a comfortable maximum and the splint is applied. Splints should be bivalved thereafter, so that physiotherapy can be given regularly. The splint is then changed every 7 to 10 days to allow a straighter cast to be applied until the objective is achieved.

Types of splints

Commoner problems are addressed through commercially made orthoses and some applications are described below.

Resting wrist and hand splints

These are made of orthoplast and are used to relieve acutely inflamed joints. They are useful as night resting splints and the wrist should be held in 10° of extension when they are applied.

Working wrist splints

The Futuro wrist splint is probably the best known in the UK. There is a metal bar on the volar surface, resting the wrist, but full use of the hand is allowed. The splint is washable and is useful in carpal tunnel syndrome and in inflammatory arthritis (Fig. 12.7). It is also prescribed in people with repetitive strain disorder, but its use here is probably unwise. An individually made orthoplast or polythene splint may be necessary if the wrist is deformed.

Working hand splints

Ulnar digital drift in rheumatoid arthritis is difficult to correct through splintage without using a cumbersome device. However, splints should be used following extensor tendon rupture in order to preserve function. An opponens

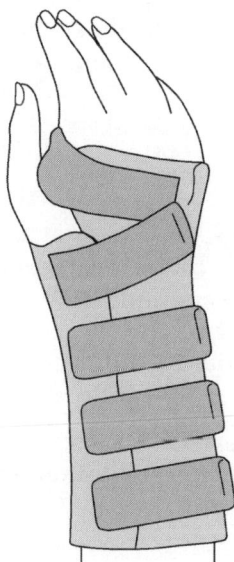

Fig. 12.7 A working wrist splint.

splint is used for the painful carpo-metacarpal joint of the thumb in generalized osteoarthritis.

Knee splints
These stabilize knees with collateral ligament or cruciate ligament dysfunction. Table 12.5 gives an indication for some of these splints.

Ankle/foot orthoses
The main indications are for foot drop following lateral popliteal nerve palsy, L5 spinal root compression, and stroke. All can be helped by an ortholon orthosis, which supports ankle and subtalar joint instability and may also incorporated insole corrections. They are lightweight and not particularly strong and cracking can occur when given severe usage by otherwise fit people or when subjected to severe spasticity. In these instances, a leg iron caliper may then be required, which is fixed to the heel of the shoe from a strap at the upper calf (Fig. 12.8).

How to get an orthosis

Footwear and orthoses can be obtained through the surgical appliance department in most hospitals and qualified orthotists are found there. Some are directly employed by

Table 12.5   Knee splints

Collateral ligament injuries:
  Mild: A simple knee corset (e.g. neoprene) allows the patient
    to exercise quadriceps and hamstring muscles.
  More severe: Hinged corset
  With deformity: Under 20° full knee orthosis
                  Over 20°—little would be of help.

Cruciate ligament injuries:
  Require more complex stabilization. Braces prevent antero-
    posterior movement.

Disrupted knees:
  Straight leg polythene jackets

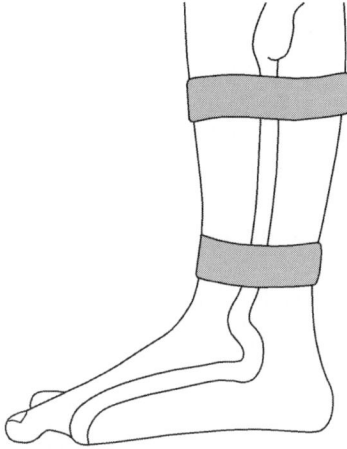

Fig 12.8 Ortholon ankle/foot orthosis.

Hospital Trusts, but others may be contracted from commercial firms. Whatever the source of the orthotist, clear benefits to patients will occur if clinicians and orthotists plan the indications and applications of orthoses for disabled people.

Prostheses

Definition

Prostheses are devices which are often implanted and which aim to substitute the control of bodily functions, which have been impaired by disease, damage, or loss. The major prostheses encountered in rehabilitation refer to artificial limbs, joint replacement, and true implanted neurological prostheses. Artificial limbs will be discussed in further detail in Chapter 25.

Joint prostheses

Joint arthroplasty has revolutionized the management of chronic joint disease. Patients can now live their lives without pain and can virtually forget the severe disability to which they were formerly subjected by their arthritis. It is useful in both degenerative (osteoarthritis) and inflammatory joint disease and most experience has been gained from hip replacement. The use of superior techniques and materials has allowed greater survival of the prosthesis and one can now expect a hip arthroplasty to last for 10 to 15 years. Results tend to be better in osteoarthritis than in rheumatoid arthritis as bone quality and the integrity of surrounding structures are more likely to be reserved. Reference to an orthopaedic or rheumatology textbook is recommended for further reading, but indications for surgery include nocturnal pain, loss of range of joint movement, such that function is impaired, progression of the underlying disease, and failure to respond adequately to medication and to physical treatment. Joint instabliity is not a contra-indication, but is likely to lead to a less favourable outcome if there is a significant deformity. Various designs of the prosthesis are now available and surgery can replace either the whole joint or part of it. Many arthroplasty prostheses are now made of a mixture of metal and plastic to reduce load and give longer life. Revision is possible if and when the prosthesis loosens, but requires great care in order to give the new artificial joint as much chance as possible of being as successful as the first. The major concern to arthroplasty operations is infection and pain in a replaced joint should alert the physician to the presence of either infection or loosening of the prosthesis. Radiographs tend not to be of much help, but occasionally sclerosis around the root of the prosthesis can indicate loosening. The investigation of choice is an isotope bone scan using technetium-99, which shows the characteristic features of loosening. If infection is suspected, gamma scanning with gallium- or indium-labelled white cells can differentiate between acute and chronic inflammation. Gallium highlights lymphocytes, whereas indium targets polymorphonuclear white cells and both are thus of great help. Infection requires prolonged antibiotic therapy for at least six to twelve weeks and may necessitate the removal of the prosthesis. The surgeon will have to be confident that infection has been irradicated before considering a new prosthesis.

Neuroprostheses

These deal with implantable devices which aim to improve functional independence and quality of life in people impaired by neurological disease, damage, or loss. They are not commonly used and therefore patients' relatives, carers, and rehabilitation professionals need to know what such devices can and cannot do. In addition, the latter need to have an understanding of the range of patients who may potentially benefit from their use. Neuroprostheses can be divided into three broad groups:

1. Substitute for lost sensory functions (sensory prostheses).
2. Substitute for lost motor functions (motor prostheses).
3. Regulate deranged sensory or motor functions (neuromodulators).

Prostheses can result in either functional neurostimulation or functional substitution. The former differs in the time domain from all other forms of medical or surgical treatment and its impact on sensory or motor function can be controlled according to the functional requirements of the moment. At present, neurostimulation is fairly crude compared with that generated by the nervous system, but is improving all the time. A report on neuroprostheses and rehabilitation has recently been published by the British Society of Rehabilitation Medicine. Neuroprostheses may for instance be able to help people considerably but do not alter the underlying impairment. They reduce disability but are not a substitute for active rehabilitation. Rehabilitation is also about education and the application of neuroprostheses must be accompanied by an educational process in their use and function. These devices are uncommon and therefore their prescription and fitting are limited to specialized centres. However, doctors referring into these centres should be certain that the present disabilities are unsatisfactorily managed and that the doctor, the patient, and the family agree that there is potential for further improvement with the use of an implant. Considerable motivation is required by some patients to gain anticipated benefits. Table 12.6 is a list of some of the devices available.

Table 12.6 Implanted neuroprostheses (after Rushden)

In use in most countries, many centres:
- Cardiac pacemakers (for cardiac arrhythmias)
- CSF shunts (for hydrocephalus)

In use in several countries, specialized centres:
- Spinal dorsal column stimulators (usually for pain)
- Phrenic stimulators (for ventilation)
- Cochlear stimulators (for profound deafness)
- Baclofen pumps (for spasticity)
- Bladder controllers (for continence and voiding)

Establishing a clinical role, more than one centre:
- Cerebellar stimulators (for spasticity, usually cerebral palsy)
- Peroneal braces (for central foot-drop)
- Activated gracilis slings (for ano-rectal incontinence)
- Upper limb stimulators (for grasps in C5/6 quadriplegia)

Investigational devices:
- Lower limb stimulators (for paraplegic standing or walking)
- Cerebellar stimulators (for epilepsy)
- Visual cortex stimulators (for blindness)
- Deep brain stimulators (for pain, tremor, or movement disorders)
- Cavernosal drug pumps (for impotence)

Environmental control systems

One of the greatest benefits that modern technology has brought to the lives of disabled people is the ability to control their own lives at home. Opening the door to a caller, closing curtains, switching channels on TV or radio seem such commonplace activities for able-bodied people, but an inability to do this can be very frustrating for disabled people. Furthermore, their carers are tied to the house and safety worries exist. Environmental control systems can change all this by providing a means for a person with a severe physical disability to control the access to his or her home, to summon emergency help, to operate everyday appliances such as the telephone, television, etc., and to switch on and off electrical power for lighting and for other pieces of equipment. Increasing independence at home means that a disabled person can do much more of what he or she wishes in safety, thereby leaving carers free to get out of the house to gain much needed respite, as well as to do the shopping, etc.

Environmental control equipment has itself considerably advanced technologically and visual display units are now commonplace. The use of radiowaves and infrared has meant that direct electrical wiring linkages between the control box and the target appliances have now disappeared, making the home much safer for the disabled individual and for carers. No longer do people have to worry about tripping over wires. In addition, whereas separate switches were required for able-bodied members of the household, this is no longer the case and they can now operate the same appliances as the disabled person, which allows better integration for all concerned.

Organizational arrangements

Environmental control systems are provided through regional centres in most parts of the country. A regional ECS coordinator is appointed to link in and liaise with local coordinators in each Health District (usually occupational therapists working within a rehabilitation centre). The regional coordinator is also responsible for training, budget management, contract negotiation, supply and maintenance of equipment, and maintenance of the contract database. The local coordinator, on the other hand, is tasked with patient follow-up, maintaining contract standards and local databases, and local liaison between users and professionals.

So how do disabled people get environmental control systems? Firstly, their attending professionals must have the training to have them in mind and know how they may be useful for a particular disabled individual. After the completed referral form is sent to the regional coordinator, a medical assessment is undertaken by a trained assessor, usually a consultant in rehabilitation medicine. The assessment includes the individual's other needs, as well as that of the environmental control system. The assessor reports back to the regional coordinator with detailed recommendations of the needs of the disabled individual and of potential solutions in the form of environmental control equipment. The client is then seen by the local coordinator, who is thereafter responsible for provision of equipment and coordination of delivery. Rehabilitation engineers assess the interface between the patient and the equipment within the home and the local coordinator will follow the individual up. Although environmental control systems are provided through the health budget, the wiring and any adaptations to the house require social services approval and funding and thus their community occupational therapists also play an important role.

The equipment

Environmental controls usually comprise three different components:
1. The selection unit, which acts as a nerve centre for the system.
2. The input from the user to control the selection or new settings for various appliances.
3. Commands to the controlled appliances.

Typical control appliances would be a door entry phone with an alarm or intercom system, light switches, telephone dialling systems, radio/TV/home entertainment control switches, and on and off facility. Curtains and doors can also be opened and closed, but are usually extra items. The switches to control systems may be operated from a wheelchair or from a static surface and various types are available. These include a hand-operated lever or joystick, a chin or headrest switch, suck and puff and pressure pad switches, as well as specialized inputs for picking up eye movements. The Steeper Fox and Possum Companion are some of the latest available models, but there are many older ones still in service, which their users find more than satisfactory.

The assessment process

What should the assessment include? The medical history and its relevance to the assessment and the cause and progress of the disabling condition are of course important. The 24 hour care profile and the hours in which a disabled person is to be left unattended must be documented. Many severely disabled people are not in fact left very much by their carers and this may be for two reasons. The first is that they do not actually wish to be left unattended and the second is that the carers are fearful of going out. Obviously, these aspects need to be tackled sensitively, but, in these circumstances an environmental control may not be very useful and may end up as yet another piece of unused equipment in the house. In addition, opportunities for socializing are important and may require inclusion in the assessment. The health and needs of the carers require documentation, along with their burden of care and any physical or lifestyle restrictions they may have. The examination should not only include the individual's motor function, but their mental state, cognitive abilities, and their special senses (vision and hearing). It is obviously important that they can see the screen or listen to the bleep sounds. Surveying the environment will inform the assessor of other pieces of equipment currently in use. Unmet needs, both social and practical, also require documentation. Armed with this information, the assessment can then recommend a particular system and a trial may be necessary in order to identify whether or not the equipment is actually appropriate and of value.

Driving

Independent mobility has transformed the lives of some disabled people and new technologies have benefitted people even with the most severe physical problems. It allows the disabled person to work, to maintain social contact and to function independently in the community. It also encourages people to communicate and raises their self-esteem. Many cars, both big and small, come as standard, with automatic transmission, power-assisted steering and with electric windows, and are more reliable and easier to drive these days.

Disabled people require information about their suitability to drive and the following questions may be addressed:

- Their safety to drive
- The most suitable type of car to acquire
- Any aids and adaptations that are required
- Sources of finance, purchase, or hire of the vehicle
- Insurance for driving and how to gain tax exemptions
- How they can stow a wheelchair if one is used
- How other people can be carried in the vehicle
- How they can be assessed by an instructor with the necessary adaptations to a learner vehicle
- Advice on alternative means of transportation if driving is not feasible.

The main medical barriers to driving are epilepsy, visual loss, cognitive deficits (in particular perceptual loss, memory loss, distraction and inattention, and intellectual loss), global dysphasia, severe mood changes, and black-outs, dizziness, etc. Loss of vision and perception mean that driving would be very difficult and it is incumbent that the rehabilitation team assesses this before raising the expectations of a disabled person to return to driving. Epilepsy is a prescribed condition for driving, for which the Department of Transport has guidelines. The ban on driving has been shortened in recent years and twelve months of freedom of seizures while awake is the norm to allow a return of a driving licence. This applies to a single fit, as well as to post-traumatic epilepsy. Nocturnal epilepsy, when seizures occur during sleep, must not have been present for three years.

Vehicle modifications

Virtually anything, it seems nowadays, can be done to a vehicle to make it suitable for a disabled person to drive. However, transportation is not only about disabled people getting behind the steering wheel. Access is also an issue. Vehicles can be adapted to allow transfer from a wheelchair to a car seat, or by build modification to allow the disabled person to travel in his or her own wheelchair in the vehicle. A whole host of seat cushions, steering aids, hand-operated controls (brakes, accelerators, etc.) can be fitted in or after manufacture so that specific adaptations do not necessarily need to be made. Certain items are now indispensible, such as a car telephone, in order to summon help quickly, if required.

Many rehabilitation centres are able to assess people on their own premises, but the Forum of UK Mobility Centres see large numbers of people. Interestingly, many otherwise able-bodied people also undertake a disabled driving assessment on their seventieth birthday in order to give them the confidence to continue driving beyond that age.

Further reading

BSRM (1994). *Prescription for independence.* A Working Party report by the British Society of Rehabilitation Medicine Enviromental Control and Special Interest Group (now the Special Interest Group on Assistive Technology). British Society of Rehabilitation Medicine, London.

BSRM (1995). *Seating needs for complex disabilities.* A Working Party report of the British Society of Rehabilitation Medicine. British Society of Rehabilitation Medicine, London. (Copies can be obtained from the Executive Secretary, BSRM c/o Royal College of Physicians, 11 St Andrew's Place, Regent's Park, London NW1 4LE, UK.)

BSRM (1997). *Neuroprostheses, neuromodulators and rehabilitation.* A report by the British Society of Rehabilitation Medicine, compiled by D. Rushden. British Society of Rehabilitation Medicine, London.

Clarke, A., Allard, L., and Braybooks, B. (1987). *Rehabilitation and rheumatology, the team approach.* Martin Dunitz, London.

Disability Information Trust (1996). *Equipment for the disabled— hoists, lifts and transfers* (and other titles). Oxford. Disability Information Trust.

Disabled Living Foundation (1994). *Handling people—equipment advice and information.* Disabled Living Foundation, London.

Fletcher, B., Holmes, D., Lloyd, P.V. *et al.* (1997). *The handling of patients* (4th edn). National Back Pain Association, Teddington.

Mulley, G. P. (1991). *Everyday aids and appliances.* British Medical Journal, London.

Mulley, G. P. (1991). *More everyday aids and appliances.* British Medical Journal, London.

Potter, R. and McLemont, E. (1997). Environmental controls. In: Goodwill, C. J., Chamberlain, M. A. and Evans, C. (ed.) *Rehabilitation of the physically disabled adult,* pp.694–705. Stanley Thornes, Cheltenham.

Section C

....

The management of
psychological disabilities

13

Behavioural problems

Staff in a rehabilitation unit often come from a background in general medicine and thus may be unfamiliar with behavioural problems. Behavioural problems in a rehabilitation unit can be poorly managed if there is limited understanding of the factors that lie behind behavioural disturbance and ignorance of potential treatment strategies. It is easy to label an aggressive individual as difficult and needing control or an individual with apathy and lack of initiation as being lazy. However, behavioural problems, particularly after traumatic brain injury or other brain insults, are remarkably common and rehabilitation staff should at least be familiar with some of the principles that lie behind behavioural management techniques. It is not possible in this chapter to cover this complex and specialist field in any detail. It is only possible to cover broad principles and give some idea of the techniques that might be helpful and benefits that might follow. Rehabilitation units which cater for individuals following brain injury must have a clinical neuropsychologist on the team and ideally should also have access to a specialist neurobehavioural unit for those individuals with severe problems.

Behavioural problems

Behavioural problems, in a rehabilitation setting, most commonly follow traumatic brain injury. However, behavioural disturbance can also follow other forms of brain insult including anoxic brain injury or occasionally in stroke or multiple sclerosis. It is also worth remembering that people with pre-existing behavioural problems secondary to mental illness or learning disabilities can also suffer a head injury and exhibit a worsening of their previous difficulty.

Behavioural problems can in general be grouped into two categories:

- inappropriate excessive behaviour
- inappropriate lack of behaviour.

The former category is more common after head injury. The most troublesome problem is usually either verbal or physical aggression. In the early stages after recovery aggression is quite common in a confused state, particularly if the individual is still in post-traumatic amnesia. As confusion settles this phase is usually followed by a general irritability which can vary from being mildly disturbed and easily contained to explosively aggressive. The more dramatic end of the spectrum is termed 'episodic dyscontrol syndrome'. Other problems of 'excessive' behaviour include difficulties with impulse control often characterized by sexual disinhibition. Typical problems that need to be managed on a rehabilitation unit are related to impulsivity, egocentrism, verbal and physical aggression, temper outbursts and socially inappropriate sexual behaviour.

At the other end of the spectrum is the individual who appears to be apathetic, lacking in initiation, and requires prompting and cajoling to undertake daily living tasks. The individual is often described as lacking in motivation. However, this is a potentially unwise label. The implication of laziness can induce a sense of therapeutic nihilism. 'It is the fault of the patient and so there is nothing we can do about it' can be readily and wrongly applied to such states.

This range of problems is remarkably common in the short term after head injury. Longer-term persistent and severe behavioural disturbance is less common and only a very small proportion of severely head injured people will need the expertise found in a specialist neurobehavioural unit.

An approach to management

Define the problem

The first question to be answered is 'what is the problem?'. The answer must be tightly defined. It is insufficient to state that 'John is aggressive'. Much more detail is needed. John may only be aggressive in particular circumstances or with particular people or doing particular things. It is usually not possible to manage a broad range of problems simultaneously and a hierarchy of importance needs to be established. For example, if a main barrier to rehabilitation is John's aggression when asked to dress in the morning then perhaps this is a good starting point for a behavioural management regime. The question 'who has the problem?' is also worth asking. Occasionally the behavioural problem in the individual is relatively mild but has a disproportionate effect on the main carer and rehabilitation staff or other people using the unit. As an example a neurorehabilitation unit admitted a gentleman with chronic schizophrenia who suffered a head injury. He had previously been in a mental institution for a number of years and was adequately managed without psychotropic medication. He always heard voices but these were usually pleasant and induced no disruptive behaviour. Occasionally the voices would tell him to walk to the other end of the hospital and sit in a sun lounge. This caused consternation amongst the nursing staff as he was rarely where he was required at times of medication or meals. Advice was sought about initiating behavioural management to keep him in the 'right' place. Once the situation was known behavioural intervention was entirely inappropriate and the nurses simply walked down the corridor to give him his tablets and remind him that it was time for his meal. Similar situations may apply in the community setting when even a relatively minor behavioural disturbance can have a disproportionate effect on marital and family relationships in an already tense situation. Sometimes a respite break or holiday is an appropriate management strategy for an apparent behavioural problem. Another relevant question is 'Who has aggravated the problem?'.

It is not uncommon in a hospital setting for disruptive individuals to be 'treated' with anxiolytics or major tranquillizers. This is nearly always unhelpful and produces additional sedation, fatigue, and clouding of consciousness. In an acute ward such intervention is occasionally required because of the danger to other vulnerable people or because more appropriate management stretches the ward resources too far. Transfer to an appropriate unit as soon as possible and cessation of such medication is the best way to manage this situation. Drug management of behavioural disturbance is further discussed below.

Study and analyse the problem

Once a problem has been identified and prioritized it is essential it is analysed in more detail. A useful approach is often described as ABC—antecedent, behaviour, consequence.

Close monitoring is required to determine the antecedent to the inappropriate behaviour. In what circumstances does it occur? What appears to trigger it? What appears not to trigger it? Is it situation specific, environment specific, person specific, or is there really no pattern discernible? What are the characteristics of the behaviour itself? For example, what form does aggression take, how long does it last and to whom or to what is it directed? Finally, what are the consequences of that behaviour? Is there obvious benefit, does it lead to a reward? Is there some form of positive reinforcement that keeps the behaviour going albeit unknown and unrecognized to the recipients?

There is normally some pattern that emerges following a period of close observation. It is often useful for such observation to be carried out quite specifically by someone who is given the task. It is often difficult to keep a close record if staff are having to do other jobs in the unit at the same time. If the problem is in the community then it is virtually impossible for a main carer to keep a dispassionate record and closely observe the behaviour pattern.

The treatment plan

Analysis of the problem and close observation over a period of time should allow for specific behaviour to be targeted. It is important to devise a measuring instrument in order to monitor whether intervention is effective. Intangible outcomes such as, 'John is less aggressive', are inadequate. Tight specific measures are required such as the number of times that John attempts to bite in a given time period at a particular time of day. Such specific goals will often require continued close observation and in turn often requires a dedicated, and trained, member of staff.

Evaluation

After a period of intervention the strategy will need to be evaluated and goals readjusted according to the outcome. Behavioural management is a dynamic phenomenon and specific goals and targets will need constant review. However, it is important to emphasize that specific behaviours can take a considerable length of time to change. More severe behavioural problems can take months under a strict regime in order to change and more particularly to generalize into other situations. There is rarely a 'quick fix' in behavioural management.

Treatment methods

This section requires a very brief overview of learning theory. This is a complex and specialist subject and this brief description will of necessity be simplistic. There are three broad areas of learning theory.

Classical conditioning
This is classical Pavlovian theory and explains behaviour in terms of learning that at least two stimuli tend to go together. In his classical experiment Pavlov demonstrated that a dog would salivate on presentation of an arbitrary stimulus such as bell or light if, on previous occasions, this stimulus had been associated with the presentation of food.

A bell or light is described as a conditional stimulus and salivation is a conditional response. This association can also be broken over time if one stimulus is not associated with the other. This break of association is called extinction. In some circumstances the association can also generalize with similar conditional stimuli, such as a different light or a bell at a different pitch.

Operant conditioning

A second theory of learning is called operant conditioning. This depends on the relationship between behaviour and the result of that behaviour. Behaviour that is closely followed by a positive result is reinforced and that behaviour is likely to be repeated. If a dog moves a lever down and receives food as a result then movement of the lever is likely to be repeated. Behaviour followed by negative effects are less likely to be repeated.

Observational or vicarious conditioning

This is where the behaviour is learnt through observation of others. A child, for example, may learn to be fearful of spiders if a parent is seen to be frightened by them.

These concepts, particularly operant conditioning, can be used to explain some aspects of post-brain injury behaviour. For example, disruptive behaviour could be interpreted in terms of the reinforcement it provides. Classical conditioning and operant condition are both forms of associative learning as they involve the formation of new linkages between one experience and another. It is known, at least in animals, that associative learning ability can be retained even in the presence of severe brain damage. Associative learning theory underlies behaviour management techniques.

Increasing desirable behaviours

Desirable behaviours can be increased in a number of ways. The commonest is by positive reinforcement. A positive reinforcer is something which is delivered following the occurrence of a behaviour which will increase the probability of that behaviour being repeated. Such reinforcers can be immediate and tangible such as food or drink, less tangible such as praise, or be a conditioned reinforcer where a person must learn the value of the reinforcement such as by receiving tokens or money. Reinforcement should be given contingently upon the occurrence of the desired behaviour—always immediately after it occurs and in a consistent and clear manner. This is vital to the success of the intervention. Other related techniques can be used. Shaping involves the reinforcement of small steps towards a desired behaviour. For example, an individual being taught to be less disinclined to dress in the mornings would be rewarded at first for looking at their clothes then perhaps touching the clothes or putting them in an appropriate place on the bed and then rewarded step by step, over a period of time, for each item of clothing that is put on. Eventually small reinforcers are withdrawn and larger steps, such as dressing the top half of the body, are reinforced until finally positive reinforcement is only received after completion of the entire task. Occasionally prompting is required and after a time the level of prompt is withdrawn (fading). Sometimes imitation of the desired behaviour is necessary by the therapist (modelling). In some centres it is possible to induce a whole token economy in which tokens are used as generalized reinforcers and can be exchanged for specific items such as extra food, drink, or social activities.

Decreasing undesirable behaviours

Various, often controversial, techniques can be used to decrease undesirable behaviours. Punishment may be used as a negative re-inforcer. 'Time-out' is a well known technique which involves withdrawal of positive reinforcement contingent upon on the occurrence of an undesirable behaviour. For example, praise may be withdrawn for a defined period of time following inappropriate behaviour, as long as praise was one of the previous positive reinforcers being used. 'Time out on the spot' involves denying attention to inappropriate behaviours such as continuing with a conversation oblivious to the behaviour or simply by walking away from the person. 'Situational time out' involves the removal of the person from the activity to another part of the room or even to a separate room for a

defined period of time. Another form of negative reinforcement is 'response cost' in which, in a token economy,
tokens are withdrawn for inappropriate behaviours as well
as being given for appropriate behaviour. Other more
controversial punishment techniques have been used
including contingent aversive stimuli which involves
unpleasant tastes or smells or even electric shocks for
undesirable behaviour. Although such techniques do
appear to work, the ethical dilemmas are obvious. Finally,
another useful technique is differential reinforcement of
other appropriate behaviour even if this is not the target
behaviour.

Overall, these techniques require a considerable amount
of skill, planning, and staff time. The techniques can take
several weeks to have an effect and can sometimes be
frustratingly difficult to generalize into a broader community setting. It is also important to emphasize that all staff
and carers involved with the individual need to be familiar
with the technique so that all behaviours are appropriately
positively or negatively reinforced. It has been thought that
behavioural management cannot be applied in the general
rehabilitation environment but some authors have demonstrated that it is possible to achieve outside a specific
neurobehavioural unit. Even in non-specialist units advice
from a psychologist can be helpful to try smaller-scale,
specific behavioural alternatives. Examples could include
training to use a toilet independently or managing to
decrease inappropriate sexual contact. Improvement in
social skills, such as joining in conversations, can also be
helped by such techniques.

Drug therapy

This chapter has strongly emphasized the value of a
psychologist to initiate a behavioural management programme. The use of sedative, anxiolytic, or psychotropic
medication is generally unhelpful and indeed may worsen
behaviour. However, in some circumstances drug treatment
of agitated behaviour can be of benefit. Indeed in some
circumstances such intervention is essential because of the
proximity of other vulnerable people or because of extreme

pressure on staff time and resources. There is little good-quality literature on this subject but some studies have indicated an improvement in aggression and episodic dyscontrol by use of the serotoninergic antidepressant, trazodone, or by use of the anticonvulsant, carbamazepine. Other authors advocate the use of lithium or betablockade with metoprolol. If severe agitation requires treatment then some would advocate the use of buspirone which is chemically distinct from other anxiolytics and is a part of class of drugs know as azapirones. For the negative behaviours some improvement is occasionally noticed following the use of dopamine agonists. A few authors have used stimulants such as dexamphetamine or methylphenidate but such medication should obviously be used with great caution and only by those with some experience in the field.

Conclusions

Behavioural disorders are common following brain injury and can be a major source of disruption to the rehabilitation programme. However, many inappropriate behaviours are amenable to behavioural management approach, albeit requiring considerable time, skill, and patience. Neuropsychologists are an essential part of a rehabilitation team. Additional support is required from a specialist neuropsychiatric behavioural unit. However, behavioural intervention can produce gratifying improvements in many people and enable them to lead a more independent life than would otherwise have been possible.

Further reading

Goldstein, L. (1993). Behaviour problems. In: Greenwood, R., Barnes, M. P., McMillan, T. M., and Ward, C. D. (ed.) *Neurological rehabilitation*, pp.389–401. Churchill Livingstone, London.

Read, A. (1997). Challenging behaviour: helping people with severe brain damage. In: Wilson, B. A. and McLellan, D. L (ed.)

Rehabilitation studies handbook, pp.263–87. Cambridge University Press, Cambridge.

Wilson, B. A. (1991). Behaviour therapy in the treatment of neurologically impaired adults. In: Martin, P. (ed.) *Handbook of behaviour therapy in psychological science*. Pergamon, New York.

14

....

Psychiatry and rehabilitation

People with physical disabilities are not immune to psychiatric problems. Conversely people with psychiatric problems are just as vulnerable as anyone else to the vagaries of life and the risk of acquiring a physical disability as a result of trauma or disease. Thus, a working knowledge of the commoner psychiatric problems is important for all members of the rehabilitation team in order to recognize when such disorders exist and initiate appropriate referrals and treatment programmes.

It is not possible nor desirable in a short chapter in this textbook to outline the whole field of psychiatry. All psychiatric conditions may be encountered by rehabilitation staff. Some conditions, such as the psychoses, clearly fall within the remit of the psychiatrist and psychotic individuals with congenital or acquired physical disabilities will nearly always need the additional assistance of a psychiatric team. Other specific conditions such as personality disorders, substance abuse, and alcoholism can often feature amongst the disabled population. People with such problems are prone to risk-taking behaviour and thus the consequent risk of trauma. Behavioural problems such as violent and antisocial behaviour or sexual disinhibition are very much part of rehabilitation practice and a good rehabilitation team should be able to make appropriate assessments and referrals for these problems. This chapter will concentrate on the recognition and management of three problems that are most commonly associated with acquired physical disability—depression, anxiety, and post-traumatic stress disorder. The chapter will not offer a definitive coverage of these fields but will attempt to highlight key factors in the recognition and treatment of these important problems.

Depression

Clinical depression is remarkably common after acquired physical disability. Depressive illness occurs in at least 50 per cent of people following stroke and severe head injury. It is almost invariable at some point during progressive neurological disabilities such as multiple sclerosis and motor neuron disease. People with congenital disabilities or disabilities acquired during childhood also have periods where they are particularly prone to depression. This is often at times of life change such as around puberty or when striving to be independent and leaving the parental home. It is often said that 'such people would be depressed wouldn't they'. It may be true that a major life change such as a serious acquired head injury is an important trigger to a depressive illness but nevertheless this should not mean that the depression should not be treated appropriately. There is no evidence that depression as a result of a physical disability responds to treatment any differently or less effectively than an endogenous depressive illness.

There is continuum of depressive illness from feeling temporarily low at one extreme to a sustained major depressive illness with suicide risk at the other extreme. Psychiatrists have invested considerable energy in drawing up specific diagnostic criteria for the classification of depression (and indeed for all other psychiatric problems). The current classification is referred to as DSM-IV (American Psychiatric Association 1994). However, there is little evidence that such classification, except in the crudest sense, is able to predict treatment response nor does classification say much about the effect of the psychiatric illness on the person's lifestyle and functioning. It is also the case that many of the psychiatric classifications are not really designed for use in people with severe physical disabilities who have a range of associated symptoms that may or may not be part of the psychiatric illness. For example, some of the categories of diagnosis of a major depressive episode include significant weight loss, insomnia, psychomotor agitation, fatigue, and diminished ability to think or concentrate. All of these problems can occur outside the context of the depressive illness in someone with a traumatic brain injury. With this caveat in mind, depressive disorders are usually characterized by sustained and depressed mood for most of the day and nearly every day. The depressed mood is normally accompanied by feelings of hopelessness or worthlessness and guilt, by behavioural problems such as social withdrawal, extreme fatigue, and crying or by biological problems such as anorexia, weight loss, insomnia, early morning waking, and loss of libido. Recurrent thoughts of death and recurrent ideas of suicide are also potentially important risk features. It is often difficult to make an assessment regarding the features that are due to depression as opposed to the physical disability, and how much the depression is actually interfering with functioning and contributing to disability and handicap. Such assessment can be triggered by a concern by the rehabilitation staff but will often need a more detailed assessment by someone with specific training in the management and assessment of mood in physically disabled people—usually a psychiatrist, psychologist, or trained counsellor.

Some units routinely administer, to those thought to be at risk, a self-rating depression scale. This can be a useful trigger to more specific assessment and intervention. Mood rating scales suffer from the problem of weighting towards biological symptoms, but despite this drawback such a screening system in a rehabilitation unit is worthy of consideration. The Hospital Anxiety and Depression Scale[1] is a good scale that excludes biological symptoms and some cognitive symptoms of depression. The Wimbledon Self-Report Scale[2] also excludes somatic items and has been developed as a suitable screening measure in a rehabilitation setting. The General Health Questionnaire[3] (28 items) is also a screening tool and is widely used in community settings and amongst general medical patients.

If intervention is required there are two broad approaches —psychological strategies and psychotropic medication.

Psychological strategies

These depend primarily on an understanding and sympathetic relationship between the counsellor or psychotherapist and the depressed individual. Information and explanation is, as always, important and can be followed by a more detailed exploration of the individual's ideas and knowledge about their illness, prognosis, the overall impact on the family, social, and work relationships, and teasing out potential stresses and coping strategies within that individual. This is good basic management and assessment which will then be supplemented by more specific counselling or psychotherapeutic approaches such as cognitive behavioural therapy, psychodynamic psychotherapy, the client centred approach of Karl Rogers, rational emotive therapy, or Gestalt therapy. The details of these different therapeutic approaches are outside of the scope of this chapter but all have enthusiastic advocates and often equally enthusiastic detractors. Counsellors or psychologists in this field often advocate an eclectic approach, individualized to that particular client.

Psychotropic medication

Medication does have an important place in the management of acute affective disorders and the prevention of recurrent problems. Lithium is the treatment of choice for bipolar disorders. However, for unipolar depressive illness there is now a wide choice of anti-depressant medication. The older tricyclic anti-depressants (such as Amitriptyline, Dothiepin, Clomipramine, and Imipramine) are good anti-depressants but are usually limited by troublesome anticholinergic side effects and sedative properties. Newer compounds such as the tetracyclic anti-depressants and the 5HT uptake inhibitors (such as Fluoxetine and Fluvox-

amine) are equally good anti-depressants with less troublesome side effects and are now generally favoured. In
specialist cases agents such as monoamine-oxidase inhibitors can be used and other types of anti-depressants such as
Carbamazepine have a place. In severe cases ECT is still a
very effective and quick anti-depressive treatment. The
treatment of severe and resistant depression is outside of
the scope of this textbook. It is worth noting that anti-
depressants should be given in a proper dosage. A positive
effect can take several weeks to be manifest and if benefit
ensues it is standard practice to continue anti-depressant
medication for at least six months.

Anxiety

Anxiety is a common companion of physical disability.
Anxiety, like depression, describes a continuum of problems and assessment will need to be made about the impact
on functional lifestyle and the necessity for intervention.
Symptoms involve a feeling of fearful anticipation, irritability, and restlessness, and worry and poor concentration.
This is often associated with physical accompaniments
including respiratory symptoms of tightness in the chest or
difficulty breathing; cardiovascular symptoms of palpita-
tions; gastrointestinal symptoms of dry mouth, difficulty
swallowing, loose bowel motions; musculoskeletal problems such as ache and tension in the scalp, neck, or
shoulders; sleep problems such as difficulty getting to sleep
and restless sleep; appetite disturbance; and central
nervous system problems such as blurring of vision,
paraesthesia, and dizziness. The individual may avoid
anxiety-provoking situations. In a rehabilitation setting
this can be interpreted as antisocial behaviour or lack of
initiation and drive.

Treatment focuses on psychological measures or medication. There are quite effective anxiety management training
programmes using a variety of approaches including
specific relaxation techniques and distraction techniques.
A variety of different counselling approaches have been
shown to be effective in controlling anxiety. If medication,

particularly sedation, is required then benzodiazepines are relatively safe and effective anxiolytics but treatment should, if possible, be short term. Withdrawal is a problem with a real risk of rebound anxiety. Anti-depressants will normally have some anti-anxiety effect, even in the absence of depression, and occasionally such medication in low doses is able to have the desired effect, with minimal side effects.

It cannot be stressed enough that anxiety, both in the disabled person and the carer and family, is often due to insufficient information and explanation about a new or worrying symptom or about the natural history and prognosis. Effective and sympathetic communication is probably the best anxiolytic.

Post-traumatic stress disorder

Post-traumatic stress disorder (PTSD) occurs after a person has been exposed to a traumatic event. The event is persistently re-experienced with recurrent or intrusive distressing recollections or dreams often as if the event were actually recurring. There is often intense distress to various triggers that symbolize or resemble part of the traumatic event. The individual will also show symptoms of stimuli associated with the trauma and a general numbing of responsiveness including efforts to avoid thoughts and feelings about the trauma and feelings of detachment or estrangement from others. There are often persistent symptoms of increased arousal, difficulty falling asleep, irritability, problems with concentration or exaggerated startle responses. It is usually considered a problem if such symptoms are present for more than a month and particularly so if the symptoms extend more than three months. Particularly after a major trauma such psychological distress can hamper rehabilitation efforts and the syndrome should be better recognized and understood by rehabilitation professionals. Obviously the syndrome can be associated with other concomitant disorders such as depression and anxiety. It seems likely that early psychological intervention produces better prognosis and thus it is important to recognize PTSD as soon as possible.

Management usually rests on psychological and psycho-therapeutic intervention rather than medication. However, for post-traumatic stress disorder couple therapy, family therapy, and in particular group therapy that helps share the experience and overcome a sense of isolation can be particularly helpful.

Conclusions

Psychiatric illness is common in a rehabilitation setting. It is important for any rehabilitation unit not to be too physically focused and to allow an environment that enables affective disorders and other potential mental illnesses to be openly discussed and accepted. Many problems can be alleviated by such an environment as well as by sympathetic sharing and giving of information and advice, particularly regarding realistic appraisal of the future. Assessment of psychiatric illness can be difficult in people with various somatic problems associated with physical disability. The need for intervention should be based on the effect on functioning and lifestyle rather than fulfilment of specific diagnostic criteria. A psychologist or counsellor with specific training in the management of psychological problems in physically disabled people should be part of a rehabilitation team and access to specialist psychiatric support is desirable. Alleviation of psychological barriers can often lead to further physical progress and improved quality of life.

References

1. Zigmond, A. and Snaith, P. (1983). Hospital Anxiety and Depression Scale. *Acta Psychiatrica Scandinvacia*, **67**, 361–70.
2. Coughlan, A. and Storey, P. (1988). The Wimbledon Self Report Scale: emotional mood appraisal. *Clinical Rehabilitation*, **2**, 207–13.
3. Goldberg, D. P. and Hillier, V. F. (1979). A scaled version of the General Health Questionnaire. *Psychological Medicine*, **9**, 139–45.

Further reading

Alexander, D. N. (1994). Depression and cognition as factors in recovery. In: Good, D. C. and Couch, J. R. (ed.) *Handbook of neurorehabilitation*, pp.129–52. Marcel Dekker, New York.

House, A. (1993). Psychiatry in neurological rehabilitation. In: Greenwood, R., Barnes, M. P., McMillan, T. M., and Ward, C. D. (ed.) *Neurological rehabilitation*, pp.403–12. Churchill Livingstone, London.

Paykel, E. S. (1995). The place of psychotropic drug therapy. In: House, A., Mayou, R., and Mallinson, C. (ed.) *Psychiatric Aspects of Physical Disease*, pp.69–78. Royal College of Physicians, London.

Rose, N. D. B. (1994). *Essential psychiatry* (2nd edn). Blackwell Science, Oxford.

15

....

Cognitive function

Cognition is a broad term that refers to all the processes involved in perceiving, learning, remembering, and thinking. These are areas that can be involved in any process that affects brain function. Traditionally neurologists and psychologists have been good at evaluating and describing such problems but not so good at actually doing anything useful about them. Recently more attention has been given to the field of cognitive rehabilitation and some progress has been made both in terms of real functional improvement and better design of coping strategies. The realm of cognitive rehabilitation has an extensive, confusing, and often contradictory literature. This chapter will not attempt to be a definitive review of this subject as this is outside the scope of the book. It will attempt to describe the extent and range of possible deficits and briefly cover some of the areas in which rehabilitation is becoming a practical possibility.

Terminology

Perceptual problems

Perception is the cognitive process that enables us to make sense of our environment. This can be through any of our senses but the most important is through our sight (visual perception), hearing (auditory perception), and touch (tactile perception). Perceptual deficits of taste and smell are described but are of less functional significance. Perception can be affected in a number of specific ways. This is a potentially confusing field and a review of commoner terminology may be helpful.

Visual agnosia is the inability to recognize objects which is not explained on the basis of a primary disorder of sensation, language, or general intellectual loss. More precise syndromes have been described including *colour agnosia* (loss of ability to recognize colours), *prosopagnosia* (loss of ability to recognize familiar faces), and *simultanagnosia* (loss of ability to perceive all the elements of a scene simultaneously and interrupt that scene—a recognition of the parts of a scene or object but not the whole). Similar problems are described such as *tactile agnosia* and *auditory agnosia*.

Related problems include *visual neglect* which is the failure to attend to one side of space or even one side of self. Such people commonly bump into things on the affected side or even fail to see food on one side of the plate thinking they have finished their meal when in fact it has only been half consumed. This problem is quite common after a stroke, particularly if the right hemisphere is involved.

Another range of perceptual problems are described as apraxias. These are conditions in which a person without general intellectual decline and without weakness, ataxia, motor defect, or defect in the sensory system is unable to execute previously learned skills and gestures. This is classically subdivided into *ideational apraxia* where there is a complete failure to conceive or formulate an action either spontaneously or on command. This has been differentiated from *ideomotor apraxia* in which the individual can know and remember the plan of action but simply cannot carry it out. There are other quite specific forms of apraxia including *constructional apraxia* which refers to problems in putting things together, such as jigsaw puzzles. *Dressing apraxia* has important functional consequences and is the inability to dress properly. Individuals would, for example, try to put on their cardigan the wrong way round or try to put on trousers upside down.

Language and communication problems

This subject is covered in more detail in Chapter 10 but it is appropriate to cover briefly some of the terminology. Problems of language are extremely common in clinical rehabilitation particularly after stroke and other focal neurological damage and disease. *Dysphasia* is the term used for language disorder which is classically divided into two types. Disorders of speech production are termed *expressive dysphasias* and disorders of comprehension are termed *receptive dysphasias*. The former is sometimes known as Broca's aphasia and the latter as Wernicke's aphasia. The dysphasias need to be differentiated from dysarthria which is a problem of the speech production itself usually due to brainstem or local mouth or pharyngeal pathology. Once again there are various defined subdisorders. Difficulty choosing the correct word is known as *anomia*. Production of an unintended or nonsense word is known as *paraphasia* and difficulty with grammar or structure of language is known as *agrammaticism*. Other specific problems include difficulty repeating despite full understanding and normal communication in other circumstances. Repetition deficits are characteristic of various *conduction aphasias*.

Often people with problems in understanding or producing speech may have associated problems with reading (*dyslexia*), writing (*dysgraphia*), and calculating (*dyscalculia*).

Memory problems

Memory is very frequently affected after any form of brain insult. It is perhaps the commonest cognitive sequela of brain injury and often one that has the most profound impact on daily function. There are many different theories and descriptors of memory deficits and a simple and practical classification is illustrated in Fig. 15.1. A distinction is usually made between short-term memory and long-term memory. The former is commonly thought to be memory over a few minutes to an hour or so. In fact short-term memory has a storage time of just a few seconds, perhaps sufficient to hold a telephone number in one's head while dialling. Long-term memory has indefinite storage time. Both long- and short-term memory seem to consist of two components—visual memory and verbal memory. Verbal memory contains all information that can be encoded into words whereas visual or visuo-spatial memory will include memory for images. The two types of memory are clearly interrelated. Memory seems to have to go through a process of encoding and storage. Longer-term memory can be split into factual storage (*declarative* memory) and storage of skills and routine (*procedural* memory). Declarative memory can in turn be split into *episodic* memory for particular events and *semantic* memory for more context-free facts. As an example remembering how to drive a car is a skill that will require procedural memory. The fact that a car is used to drive one to work could be described as semantic memory, and the fact that the car was actually used to drive to work that morning is an episodic memory. Finally, stored memories will obviously need to be retrieved and used at the appropriate time. It is likely that these different memories are served by different neural circuits, although clearly there is a very close interrelated network.

Memory disorders are generically called amnesias. The term *retrograde amnesia* is usually associated with a cerebral injury and applies to the loss of memory prior to the injury. This is usually a very short spell. *Anterograde amnesia* refers to ongoing memory disturbance after a particular event. The commonest is *post-traumatic amnesia* which describes the period of time after cerebral insult before continuous day-to-day memory re-occurs.

Attention and other problems of higher executive function

Attention is the ability to remain aware of our surroundings. It is also the ability to selectively attend to particularly important signals. For example, one may be listening to music and can divert attention if someone starts a conversation although the music is still playing. Various problems with attention can clearly result in daily living difficulties. Classically after brain injury a number of attention deficits can be found. Brain injured people can have problems with selective attention and find it difficult

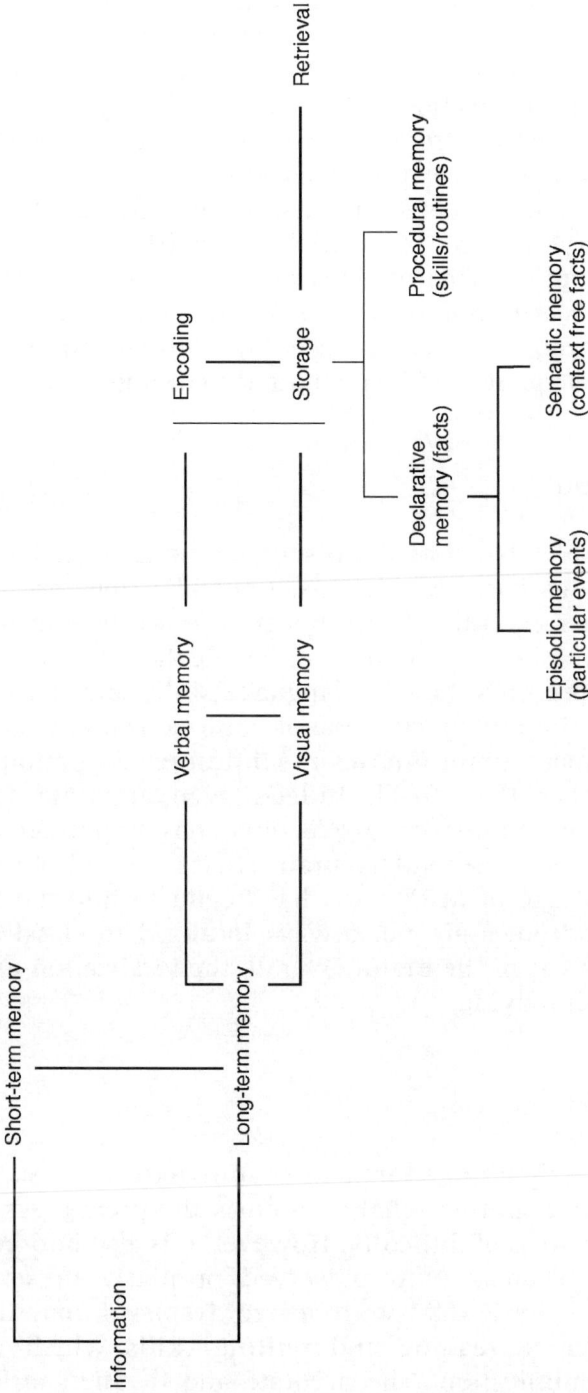

Fig. 15.1 Long and short term memory.

to exclude the less important inputs. At a party, for example, they may not be able to selectively attend to the person with whom they are talking if there are other background conversations. They may also have problems in alternating attention from one task to another such as when driving a car, or have problems with dividing attention to respond simultaneously to two or more things at once, such as carrying on a conversation while driving. Typically in brain injury other problems arise that are often called deficits in *higher executive function*. These include such difficulties as problem solving, reasoning, putting actions into the correct sequence, judgement, and planning.

Localization

I have completely avoided a discussion on the localization of the various cognitive deficits. Generalizations are possible. Higher executive functions are classically associated with frontal lobe damage. In most people the left side of the brain is more important for language skills and the right side more important for spatial and perceptual skills. However, many brain injuries in clinical rehabilitation are diffuse rather than focal. Indeed even apparent focal damage from trauma or stroke often has important and more widespread secondary brain effects. In addition the widespread use of MRI scans has begun to indicate that precise syndromes are not always localized to classically described areas of the brain. Overall, the localization game is not worth playing.

Assessment

There is clearly a huge range of cognitive difficulties. The first task in cognitive rehabilitation is the precise assessment of the areas of difficulty. However, it is also important to document areas with preserved or partly preserved function. An individual with severe dysphasia may have some preserved reading and writing skills which will allow communication. The accurate and detailed task of cognitive assessment lies within the realm of the clinical neuropsychologist who is thus an essential part of the neurological rehabilitation team.

Cognitive rehabilitation

Is it possible to restore cognitive function? This is a controversial question with little definitive evidence of an answer. Studies are fraught with difficulties and natural recovery clearly needs to be differentiated from recovery through a rehabilitative programme. Classical placebo-controlled, double-blind studies are almost impossible in this field and progress will rely on single-case methodology. There is some evidence through such methodology that indicates attentional deficits can be improved as can some cases of unilateral neglect and some deficits in communication, including dyslexia.

Whilst, however, restoration of function is difficult to achieve there can be significant functional benefit from a broad cognitive rehabilitation approach. Two broad approaches are possible:

- bypass the problem or find another way to achieve the same goal
- use residual skills more effectively.

Finding a way around the problem

A number of strategies can be adopted. Individuals can be provided with assistive equipment. People with memory problems can be taught to use external memory aids such as diaries, lists, alarm clocks, timers, or tape recorders. This is not always successful as individuals need residual memory in order to remember what they are being reminded about! However, there are commercial systems that are radio controlled and a central switchboard will transmit a message into a small 'bleeper' screen. In other circumstances it is possible to rearrange the immediate environment in order to reduce the need for cognition. Rigid organization is sometimes required for those with disordered organizational skills. A very structured day helps people to cope with difficulties with planning. Organization of physical space, such as labelling drawers, can also be helpful. Occasionally more dramatic labelling of the environment is required such as colour-coded doors or different coloured lines on the floor in order to guide the person from, say, the bedroom to the toilet. Sometimes very simple measures can help such as supplying simple clothing with velcro fastening for people with mild forms of dressing apraxia. A whole variety of strategies are possible often needing not just an accurate neuropsychological assessment but an application of common sense and lateral thought.

Using residual skills more effectively
Techniques in this area have been mainly developed in the field of memory. Mnemonic strategies have been used including imagery where information is remembered by an association with a particular image. An example is the PQRST mnemonic. In this technique individuals are taught to Preview information, set Questions to themselves on the information, Read information over, State the information again, and Test the results. This is really an enlargement of a repetition strategy by which it is hoped that information is 'deeper' encoded. Other techniques can make use of acronyms, rhymes, and systematic cueing where a well known series such as an alphabet is scanned through to cue an appropriate memory. This, and other, techniques designed to use residual skills more efficiently, have been clearly shown to produce real functional benefit and lessened disability in many individuals. Approaches are by no means mutually exclusive and different strategies can be employed simultaneously in the same person.

As always it is important to involve the carer in planning the strategy as all those who come into contact with the individual must be aware of the problems and act accordingly and in line with the strategic goals and plans.

Conclusions

There are a great variety of cognitive problems that can arise within the context of neurological disability. A full assessment is essential in order to clearly identify problems as well as identifying residual areas of strength and preserved function. There is now emerging evidence that cognitive rehabilitation can in certain, but still limited, circumstances restore at least some function. However, if this is not possible then coping strategies can often be designed which bypass the problem or use residual or alternative skills more effectively. In every case, even if rehabilitation is not possible for a particular cognitive difficulty, assessment, information, and explanation is essential. Such information must be imparted if at all possible to the disabled person as well as the carer and family. An understanding of the problem can itself lead to improved function and certainly less risk of unnecessary worry and anxiety.

Further reading

Hardin, L. and Beech, J. R. (ed.) (1996). *Assessment in neuropsychology*. Routledge, London.

Lezak, M. D. (1995). *Neuropsychological assessment* (3rd edn). Oxford University Press, Oxford.

Wilson, B. (1987). *Rehabilitation of memory*. Guildford Press, New York.

Wilson, B. and Moffat, N. (1992). *The clinical management of memory problems* (2nd edn). Chapman and Hall, London.

Wood, R. L. L. and Fussey, I. (ed.) (1990). *Cognitive rehabilitation in perspective*. Taylor and Francis, London.

Section D

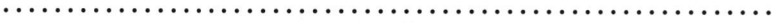

Handicap

16

··

Broader issues in rehabilitation—handicap and participation

Rehabilitation of the disabled person involves minimization of disability and handicap. However, a clinical rehabilitation team will mainly concentrate on the former rather than the latter. Handicap factors are often outside the control of health professionals. Naturally the team will develop strong liaison with other professionals who can assist with the reduction of handicap. Professionals from employment rehabilitation services, education services, and, in particular, the local authority departments such as social services and housing have a major role to play in this sphere. Other factors are outside the control of even the broader rehabilitation team and lie within the realms of societal attitudes and government legislative policy. However, it is vital for a clinical rehabilitation team to have a grasp of handicap issues. This chapter will briefly outline some of the key topics that will need to be addressed in order that minimum disability can be put into the context of minimum handicap. Details of organizations and legislation will clearly vary considerably from country to country. It is not possible to make meaningful and broad statements in this context. Thus, this chapter has a UK orientation but it is hoped that some of the principles involved are applicable regardless of geographical location. It is also clear that much of the content of this chapter depends on legislation which can also change. It is likely this chapter will date quite quickly but it was felt helpful to include an overview of the present situation in the UK to give some idea of the issues involved and areas in which new legislation may be useful. The areas to be addressed are:

- education and further education
- school leavers
- employment
- housing and home adaptations
- leisure interests
- finance and benefits
- legal problems
- carers.

Education and further education

Children with disabilities in the UK have to remain in an educational environment at least until the age of 16 years. In the last 20 years there has been some improvements in the educational provision for disabled children. Baroness Warnock produced a government report in 1978 which was critical of a number of aspects of education, in particular the requirements of those with special needs. The report was followed by the 1981 Education Act which required an assessment of special needs to be recorded in a document called a Statement. The details of procedures and appeals have been further enshrined in the 1993 and 1996 Education Acts. The Statement is an assessment of special education requirements and is usually a multidisciplinary process made not only by teaching staff but by educational psychologists and, if necessary, therapists and physicians. The Statement has to be agreed by the parents and has to be reviewed annually. The Statement at least provides a framework for the rehabilitation programme. However, resources within the education sector rarely match required needs and inadequacies of service provision still exist.

Historically there has been a tendency to keep disabled children in special and separate educational provision.

However, in recent years there has been a trend away from special school provision towards the integration of disabled children into mainstream schooling. Although this trend is to be encouraged there are undoubtedly problems, particularly if adequate resources do not follow the child. Many mainstream school buildings are inaccessible for those with special needs, particularly those with wheelchair requirements. There may be inadequate specialist teachers for the large number of mainstream schools. Children can be cruel, and some studies have demonstrated that disabled children can be more isolated amongst able-bodied peers than with disabled school friends. Special schooling does have the advantage of physical accessibility and the ability to provide a range of specialist teaching staff. However, the traditional view of special schools is that they cater for a broad intellectual range and do not cater well for physically disabled children without intellectual problems. There are clearly arguments in favour of both mainstream and special school provision. Much of the argument hinges on the adequate resourcing of special needs teaching.

Many disabled children will have congenital disabilities but the specific problems of children who acquire disabilities should not be forgotten. Such children will often have been brought up within mainstream school with able-bodied friends. They may have great difficulty in re-integration or may have both physical and intellectual problems which make it difficult to relate to their own friends and may be well behind in schooling and have to face the problem of going down a class or having special tuition. Such children will clearly need sensitive handling and the rehabilitation team will often need to invest considerable time in liaison with the school, hospital teaching staff, educational psychology services, and the Local Education Authority.

Students with disabilities often need extra time to obtain appropriate educational goals. They may have learning disabilities or may have had considerable time in and out of hospital or time out of the classroom for therapy sessions. The need for extra years in education for disabled youngsters has been recognized in the Further and Higher Education Act 1992 which gives the opportunity for education up to

25 years old. Such provision clearly depends on both funding opportunity and the availability of an appropriate school or college. Most further education will take place in the sixth form attached to a school but is now becoming as commonly provided in a Further Education College. Such colleges tend to concentrate more on newer vocational qualifications whereas school sixth forms tend to concentrate more on academic qualifications leading to university places. However, this distinction is becoming more blurred with time. The disabled youngster has an additional, albeit limited, option of attending some of the residential training colleges which are able to deliver individual programmes, particularly to those with more severe disabilities. When children are striving to gain independence a time away from home in a residential college is worth considering. There is an increasingly confusing array of vocational and academic courses on offer for the 16–19 year old. Advice should be obtainable from the school careers service or more specifically from a specialist careers adviser who is usually employed by the Local Education Authority specifically to advise disabled youngsters.

At higher education level there is even more choice of courses. The student will often need advice not only on the choice available and whether they will obtain the necessary academic qualifications but also on the accessibility of the university campus itself. Many older universities are virtually inaccessible for wheelchair users. Universities vary enormously with regard to provision for disabled students and an actual visit to view accommodation and teaching areas and discuss particular requirements with lecturing staff is to be encouraged.

Finance at university can be a problem. Local Education Authorities are responsible for grants for most higher educational courses although awards are usually means tested and a contribution is often required from parents or spouses of students under 25 years of age. However, there are some other sources of funding including further discretionary awards from the Local Education Authority and other discretionary awards from the Further Education Funding Councils. There are other awards available including disabled students allowances and various forms of student loans. The situation can be complicated and advice from the University, specialist careers adviser or from Skill (National Bureau for Students with Disabilities) is advisable. The latter organization publish a useful range of information sheets for students with disabilities.

Finally, the rehabilitation team should not forget that disabled adults are able to access higher education. Many with acquired physical disability can usefully retrain or learn new skills through the higher educational sector. The increasing availability of distance learning packages through, for example, the Open University, as well as a number of evening, weekend, or residential courses, do now provide a large range of educational opportunities. The Local Education Authority and local university or college should be able to provide details of the course and details of accessibility, flexibility, and suitability for the potential student.

Transition to adult life—the disabled school leaver

During their childhood years, people with disabilities have had fairly well coordinated services from health, educational, and social services, but organizational changes occur after their sixteenth birthday which diminishes their potential for independence. Paediatricians tend to cease their input at around this time and educational input changes as children leave school and either take up further education or seek employment. Slightly later on, social services responsibilities, as defined by the Children's Act 1991, end and they move into adult disability care. As a result, new teams of professionals appear for the provision of social care and rehabilitation and the result of all this can be confusing thereby losing young people with disabilities to follow-up.

Adolescence is also a time of great personal change, both for young people themselves (and we all remember how difficult adolescence can be!), as well as for families. Difficulties can be magnified in the presence of a chronic disability and, as a result, many young people do not realize their ambitions through a lack of knowledge of what is available to help them and through diminished and inequitable access to opportunities for independent living. This applies to all disabled young people and it is known that the families of those with congenital disabilities and those who have been disabled from a very early age, have far lower expectations for the young person than those with relatively newly acquired functional loss. On top of this, these young people have a poor self-image thereby accentuating their dependence. Parents are often unwilling to let their disabled child try to be independent and services mismatch individuals' needs. A survey in Gloucestershire in 1988 highlighted this and the main elements of the subsequent report (Beardshaw 1988) are listed below:

1. A lack of a coordinated rehabilitation service.
2. A shortage of skilled specialists in social services and health.
3. Poor liaison between services leading to fragmented services to clients.
4. Lack of readily available information resource for service users and for providers.
5. Inadequate provision of certain services.
6. Inadequate provision and lack of choice of residential accommodation.
7. Inadequate day care provision outside city centres.

So what are the main issues facing disabled young people as they leave school? Hardoff and Chigier (1991) identified that the main developmental tasks in the transition from puberty to the middle of the third decade in life are for people to consolidate their identity, achieve independence of parents, establish adult relations outside the family, and find a vocation. Young people therefore need many skills and disabled people are often at a disadvantage when compared with their able-bodied peers. They have often missed out on a wide variety of essential experiences, perhaps because of a lack of independent mobility, but very often due to a lack of financial independence and independence from parents.

The health problems facing disabled adolescents

So what are the problems that confront young people as they leave paediatric care? Many will be related directly to their underlying conditions. Spasticity and athetosis in cerebral palsy, for instance, can be quite disabling and obviously the combination of physical and learning disabilities will have a huge impact on the life of the young person and his or her family. People with spina bifida have difficulties related not only to their mobility, but to tissue viability and to renal function. However, there are some areas of health deficiency, which are common to most young people with disabilities. They have trouble accessing their general practitioner or their dentist and there is an increased incidence of visual acuity problems, of orthopaedic problems, of problems with their feet and with their dental hygiene. In addition, there is an increased incidence of pressure sores, contractures, and incontinence and they are very often under weight. Respiratory difficulties, particularly recurrent chest infections, can occur in people who have truncal weakness, because of developing scoliosis and fixation of the chest. All the above lead to a failure to thrive, which is essential for maturation to adulthood. Similarly, cognitive and behavioural impairments also diminish maturation and the whole is made worse by the effect on personal esteem due to skeletal deformities. Multiple problems are common and it is important to be able to assess whether the combination of these has an additive effect on the ability to learn new tasks.

However, most important are the constraints placed on young people with physical disabilities, as they attempt to find their way in the world. Choosing a career and a lifestyle is difficult for all of us, but for young people with physical disabilities, it is even harder. Some of the constraints are described in Table 16.1 and the effect of service mismatching or of a lack of knowledge of what is available often leads to the impression that nobody cares.

Epidemiology

How big is the problem? Table 16.2 shows the relative incidence and prevalence of some of the more common conditions. In service provision terms, cerebral palsy itself makes up the largest group of young people presenting

....

Table 16.1   Constraints on disabled young people

Constraint	Examples
Resources	Lack of appropriate facilities
Personal ability	Low self-esteem and self-image
Family concern	Letting go of childhood
Service mismatching	Failure to match client with facility

(about one-third). Spina bifida still produces significant numbers, but fortunately the trend is now reducing. Neuromuscular rarities together form a significant group presenting with common features and common needs. Cystic fibrosis, for instance, used to result in significant mortality before the age of 16 years, but recent advances have improved not only the survival, but the quality of life for these young people. Disabled young people aged between 16 and 29 years, constitute about 5 per cent of all disabled people and 2.5 per cent of the population in this age group. This calculates at some 340 000 young people, of whom 20 000 are living in residential care or in communal establishments. More than half of this disabled population have a very severe disability in category 7 or above of the OPCS Scale.

Requisite skills for adolescents

In order to be of assistance to these young people, it is necessary to identify the requisite skills required to make a successful transition from childhood to adolescence (Table 16.3).

Service provision

What does this group of young people need from statutory services? Some of the main issues are listed below:
- Health care and personal issues (disability, psycho-sexual, genetic counselling)
- Aids and equipment for daily living, education, and employment

Table 16.2 Incidence and prevalence of some diseases seen in young adults

Disease/injury	Incidence per 10^6	Prevalence per 10^6	Prevalence trend
Congenital			
Cerebral palsy	200		Static
Spina bifida	Variable	2	Down
Muscular dystrophy—all types	1–3/8000 live births	90	Down
Neurological rarities	Make large group together		Down
Cystic fibrosis	40/2500 live births		Increasing in over 15-year-olds
Acquired			
Head injury	300	150	Up
Spinal injury	1015		Static
Juvenile chronic arthritis	16	Up to 113	Static
Multiple sclerosis	48	99178	Static

Table 16.3 Skills required of young adult

	Maintenance skills				Life skills		
	Self-care	Domestic	Mobility	Relationships	Leisure	Work	Self-development
Health	Feeding	Food collection, preparation, storage	Indoors	Sexual	Hobbies	Direct work skills and mobility to work and within workplace	Assertiveness
Nutrition	Dressing	Maintenance of clothes	Threshold	Family			
Exercise	Hygiene	Home cleaning/maintenance	Outdoors	Social	Sport	Posture and seating	Negotiation
Disease management		Home safety	On foot/in wheelchair, using transport, public/private	Work			Time management
Disability management							Money management
Use of NHS resources (e.g. GP, dentist)		Money management		Community			Information gaining
				Other			Career development

- Information
- Independent living skills
- Social needs, personal care, finance, and occupational activity
- Further education and training
- Employment
- Transport/mobility/access
- Housing
- Leisure and recreation facilities.

Service provision can be related to the principal pathologies, as in cerebral palsy, spina bifida, or juvenile arthritis, or it can be provided as a specialized integrated service. Multiprofessional Young Adult Teams are now well established in certain parts of the United Kingdom. Some also have an input from education and social services and teams exist which deal purely with the social and educational needs of young people. The voluntary sector is extremely valuable in this area of work, as they hold a huge information resource, which is particularly useful to young people. Most service models are multidisciplinary in nature and some of the participants in such a team could be as follows: doctor with rehabilitation expertise; physiotherapist; occupational therapist; speech and language therapist; social worker; clinical psychologist; nurse; specialist careers officer; secretary; links with housing and with voluntary sector/disability organizations etc.

Young Adult Teams have many links with statutory and voluntary organizations, and Fig. 16.1 shows their relationships. These form a mixture of well-established linkages such as between rehabilitation services and wheelchair services, whereas others require specific working in order to ensure contact between the various players. It is obviously important to have a full range of services for the client group which by and large span the age group from 16 to 25 years or 30 years and to teach them how to maintain their skills and how to seek help should their situation change. Rehabilitation for these people is a lifelong process and contact during adolescence should not be left without follow-up. This implies a burden on statutory services, but the cost of responding as an emergency to unmet needs later on in life is actually greater than in dealing with life events in a proactive way. The key to this follow-up is good communication between the young people, the young adult team and the general practitioner. The latter's importance in this role cannot be under-estimated, as it is known that young people are twice as likely to require face to face contact with their GP than their able-bodied peers.

Successful services are based on a philosophy which responds to the needs of clients and allows them to realize their ambitions and acquire the necessary skills for the future. The aim is in enhancing personal control of situations and therefore in achieving independence. Informed choice is a key to successful integration of disabled people (and of able-bodied people as well) and the Living Options principles (Prince of Wales Advisory Group 1985) has been widely accepted in the United Kingdom. The disabled person's aims for choice, consultation, participation, recognition, information, and autonomy are sacrosanct.

Employment

Disabled people have very high rates of unemployment. However, only very few people with the most severe

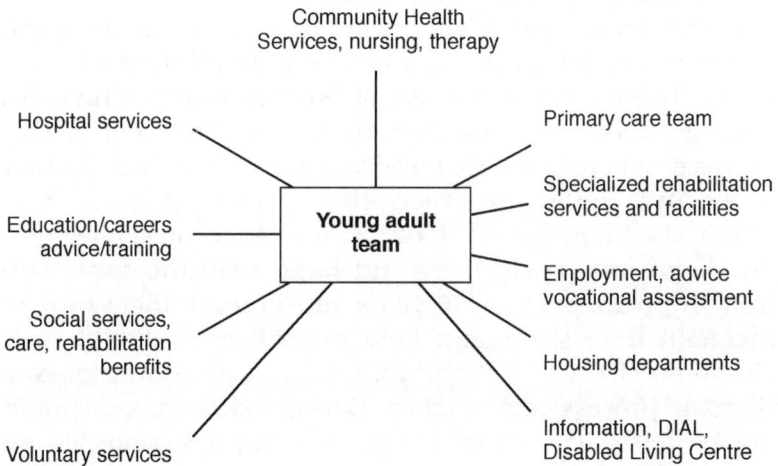

Fig. 16.1 Links with services.

physical and cognitive problems are totally incapable of work. In many cases unemployment is a result of lack of information, either by the disabled person who has not been made aware of employment opportunities or by potential employers regarding the effects of a particular disability on work performance. The situation is compounded at times of high unemployment when an employer often has a number of able-bodied job applicants and is unlikely to take on the additional perceived risks of employing a disabled person. Traditionally there is very little contact in the UK between the clinical rehabilitation team and the employment rehabilitation service. The two services are the responsibility of different government departments and there is little formal interchange between them. Cooperation and mutual understanding often depend purely on local contacts and goodwill. This is surprising when studies looking at the overall cost of disability to the State confirm that most of the cost relates to lost employment opportunities, and the consequent need for State support. It has, for example, been estimated that the annual cost of multiple sclerosis in England and Wales is £125 million at 1986 prices. £100 million of this figure represented lost earnings and thus only 20 per cent represented the cost of consultations, prescriptions, hospital, and community care.

Under the new UK Disability Discrimination Act 1995 it is unlawful to treat a disabled person less favourably than someone else because of their disability unless discrimination is 'justified'. Furthermore employers must also take reasonable steps to prevent their practices or premises from causing substantial disadvantage to the disabled person. This legislation should help to reduce discrimination in the workplace.

What can be done? First, the rehabilitation team must be familiar with the employment rehabilitation system. The key local person is the Disability Employment Adviser (DEA) who will work with the disabled person to assess abilities and disabilities and offer practical advice and assistance in finding a suitable vacancy. The DEA is a member of PACT (Placing, Assessment, and Counselling Team) who can offer more detailed assessment and advice. The teams are mobile and are able to visit employers and employees within the work place. This can be useful for those with acquired disabilities who may wish to return to their old job. Various grants are available for employers to help adapt the workplace. This can range from ramps at an entrance, adapting an existing toilet to make it wheelchair accessible, purchasing specific office furniture, and helping with the purchase of specialist equipment. If further training is required this can be organized at the local Ability Development Centre (ADC) or can be subcontracted elsewhere.

Training for work is now the responsibility of Training and Enterprise Councils (TECs). TECs can provide Youth Training which is available for all younger people under the age of 18 but special arrangements are available for disabled youngsters who are guaranteed a place after 18 if their disability prevented earlier entry providing they are able to complete training before they are 25. Modern Apprenticeships also offer training to school leavers but usually to a slightly higher standard than the YT schemes. Training for Work schemes are also available for long-term unemployed people but disabled people do not have to satisfy the usual requirement of being unemployed for six months. Training for Work is available as residential training in 16 residential training colleges around the UK for people with severe disabilities or special local training can be arranged by the TEC with extra funds from the Department for Education and Employment. Residential training is now managed by the Residential Training College Unit based in Newcastle upon Tyne.

Problems for many disabled people are not only related to finding a job but to retaining it. This is particularly true for individuals with more subtle higher executive dysfunctions such as with problem solving, organizational planning, sequencing, and skills of social interaction. Such problems can be dealt with by information and explanation to the employer and work colleagues. A scheme in the United States, Job Coach, provides for a skilled worker to be alongside the disabled person in the early days of employment to help iron out difficulties and misunderstandings and to further the training and rehabilitation of the individual within the real world. Such schemes have quite high success rates both in terms of employment and job retention.

Employment offers many opportunities for the application of new technology. This is particularly true for computer and communication technology. Physical workplace problems will often need one-off solutions and the skills of the clinical team and a rehabilitation engineer can be useful.

Flexibility is important. For some disabled people full-time employment on the open market is a possibility. However, for many part-time flexible working is necessary. Others will need relatively simple tasks in a sheltered and structured environment. Some opportunities are still available in various sheltered workshops but such facilities tend to suffer from boring and demeaning contract work and poor pay. Some more enlightened disabled employers have now entered the market. There are a number of successful businesses run for or by disabled people. In and around Newcastle upon Tyne, for example, such businesses include garden furniture manufacturing, printing, market gardening, and desk-top publishing. The advent of distance computer working can also allow many disabled people to work from home. The Employment Service now runs a Supported Employment Programme specifically designed to help people with severe disabilities who are unlikely, because of their limited productivity, to get and keep jobs in open employment without some support. It offers many kinds of job opportunities from catering and office services to manufacturing and horticulture. Employment is sponsored through voluntary bodies, local authorities, and Remploy (a government sponsored private company) in special workshops and factories or in supported placements in firms.

There are now a number of financial incentives for employers to take on disabled people as well as financial assistance to the disabled person. Job Introduction Schemes are available to all disabled people who may require a period of adjustment in a job and demonstrate their capabilities to a new employer. The Employment Service will pay a sum to a firm if it agrees to give a six week trial to the disabled person. Access to Work is a programme that can assist with extra costs involved in: employing a communicator for people who are deaf or have a hearing impairment; a part-time reader for someone with impaired vision; support workers if practical help is needed at work or getting to work; special equipment or adaptations; alterations to premises; and help with travel to work costs such as adaptations to a car or taxi fares.

The Disability Working Allowance is a tax-free sum paid on top of low wages. The allowance is intended to encourage people with disabilities to return to work by topping up low earnings. The rules are complex and not entirely without controversy. Details of this and other allowances are available from the Disability Advice Centre or are summarized in the useful Disability Rights Handbook (see Further Reading).

Traditionally the employment rehabilitation service has concentrated on the retraining of those with relatively minor physical problems such as back pain. Training and expertise amongst employment rehabilitation staff is less concentrated on the problems of those with severe physical and cognitive disabilities. The assessment skills of a neuropsychologist or rehabilitation physician are rarely available to the employment team. Improved training for the employment rehabilitation team and improved awareness of employment opportunities by the health team as well as mutual cooperation and communication are essential in order to maximize employment opportunities for disabled people.

Housing and home adaptations

Housing in the UK is generally inadequate for disabled people. Steps to the front and back door are common, doorways are narrow and awkward for wheelchairs, and toilets and bathrooms are often inaccessible and usually upstairs. A home visit by an occupational therapist, often with a counterpart in the social services department, is an important early step in the rehabilitation process. Delays in housing adaptations are the commonest cause of delays in discharge from hospital.

Sometimes relatively simple adaptations are all that are required. Judicious use of grab rails, a raised toilet seat, a sliding board to access the bath, or a simple ramp to the front door may be all that is needed. More complex adaptations such as widening of doors, provision of wheelchair accessible showers, ceiling hoists, stair-lifts, or through floor lifts may be necessary but unfortunately often prone to the long process of assessment, approval, and provision by the local authority social services and housing departments. Disabled facilities grants (Housing Act 1996 and Housing Grants, Construction and Regeneration Act 1996) are paid by local housing authorities on both a mandatory and discretionary basis to help disabled people with the cost of home adaptations. All grants are means tested and payable up to a maximum of £20 000. Recent legislation does allow authorities discretion to pay above this limit in certain circumstances. Unfortunately this system is somewhat complicated and the assessment, approval, and implementation process can take many months. It is possible that the system will change at the time of writing due to a change of government and up-to-date advice should be obtained from the local housing department or disability advisory centre.

Unfortunately for some people there is little alternative but to move house. In many countries, particularly Scandinavia, there is a broad range of disability housing. However, the situation in the UK is less encouraging. Some housing developers build a proportion of houses suitable for wheelchairs. Other possibilities are various forms of sheltered housing that have wardens or other personal care services as an integral part of the community. In some parts of the country there are separate village communities of disabled people with full adapted housing and mutual support networks. However, such possibilities are unusual in the UK and regrettably the more severely disabled person is quickly faced with the prospect of admission to either a residential or nursing home. There is an increasing choice of such homes within the private sector but nevertheless it is unfortunate that the step from living at home to living in an institution is the reality of choice for many disabled people. It should not be forgotten that disabled people will occasionally make a positive choice to live in an institution. This is particularly so for more severely disabled people without a partner or carer who value the daily contact with other disabled people and care staff. The provision of residential placement is usually coordinated by the local authority who now have an obligation to ensure that a high proportion of such housing is provided through the private sector. More severely disabled people with ongoing health requirements are the additional responsibility of the National Health Service and indeed some residential units are an integral part of the hospital or rehabilitation unit.

Accessible and appropriate housing is an obvious, essential pre-requisite for the disabled person to live within the community. It is a pity that many disabled people are faced with little or no choice with regard to housing. There is an urgent need for a broader range of housing opportunities.

Leisure interests

Able-bodied people follow a variety of hobbies, sports, and other pastimes. Unfortunately many leisure opportunities are not available to disabled people. The loss of a previous interest combined with concomitant loss of friends has a major emotional impact on the disabled person. This is particularly so if the person also has increased leisure time available because of the restrictions placed on mobility or work. An assessment of leisure interests by the rehabilitation team is essential part of the rehabilitation process. It will enable, if at all possible, a suitable programme to be developed that is of some relevance and interest to the person. For example, a young man with a passion for computer games cooperated in therapy sessionsonly when he was allowed to finish the session with a brief spell of computer games. His interest in computers eventually extended to desk-top publishing skills and the establishment of his own business. A head injured young lady with a previous interest in art responded well to a programme that enabled her to draw in a variety of environments both within and outside the rehabilitation unit.

There are a number of sports and hobbies that remain accessible to disabled people and can provide much entertainment, occupation, and pleasure. There are many active sports that can be enjoyed including wheelchair basketball, wheelchair abseiling, rally driving, and flying. Obviously there are quieter interests such as wheelchair dancing, angling, and computing. The pursuit of hobbies often just requires some mutual assessment of residual skills and interests combined with a local knowledge of suitable clubs and societies, including able-bodied clubs that allow physical accessibility. There are some centres that offer the opportunity for disabled people to try out various outdoor activities such as the Calvert Trust centres in Northumberland, Cumbria, and Devon.

The need for holidays is also important as a break for the disabled person, carer, and family, either together or separately. There are now a number of specialist holiday companies that cater for disabled people and can supply suitable venues and accessible hotels. Public transport can remain a problem. Airlines can be helpful given notice in order to provide transport at the terminal and help on and off the aircraft. Rail travel can still be difficult but is improving in terms of accessibility. The local disability advice centre should be able to provide assistance and literature on a wide range of leisure interests and holiday opportunities.

Finance and benefits

Disability is expensive. First, many disabled people have a low income from being unemployed, being forced to take part-time employment or employed in more menial and lower paid tasks. Second, outgoings are increased because of the costs of disability such as equipment, increased clothing needs, increased heating costs, contribution to housing adaptations, travel costs to hospital, and a whole variety of other expenditure. Other sections of this chapter and other parts in the book have highlighted some of the financial support that is available. Regrettably the social security benefit system and the range of benefits from local authority and other sources is extremely complicated. Many studies have demonstrated that few disabled people receive all the benefits and grants to which they are entitled. The rehabilitation team has an obligation to have a working knowledge of the major benefits and should have access to a disabled advice centre, welfare rights centre, or a social worker who can go through all entitlements and make sure that all support is accessed. It is not possible in this chapter to outline the whole range of benefits which in any case change with rapidity, particularly after a change of government. The reader is referred to the Disability Rights Handbook which is published by the Disability Alliance each April and is a very useful guide to benefits and services available to disabled people and their carers.

A few broad and important headings will be covered.

Inability to work

If previously in employment a newly disabled person is entitled to Statutory Sick Pay for 28 weeks after which Incapacity Benefit is payable. If the person has not made sufficient National Insurance contributions for incapacity benefit and is at least 80 per cent disabled or incapable of work since before the age of 20 Severe Disablement Allowance is currently payable. If none of these are available or if total income is still insufficient to live on then individuals can apply for Income Support. Disabled people who are unemployed but are capable of some form of work are entitled to a Job Seekers Allowance which has recently replaced Unemployed Benefit and Income Support for certain categories of individuals capable of work. A Disability Working Allowance is a tax-free allowance paid on top of low wages or self-employed earnings for people with disabilities that put them at a disadvantage in getting a job. The qualifications and amount of the allowance as well as necessary claim, payment, and appeal procedures are complicated but the additional income obtained does allow a number of disabled people to get back to work, albeit often in rather menial and low-paid jobs. It is one small way of getting out of the 'benefit trap' which makes it very difficult for many disabled people to actually be better off working than remaining unemployed.

Care needs and mobility problems

The Disability Living Allowance (DLA) is a benefit for people with disabilities and primarily aimed at those who need some help to look after themselves or people who find some difficulty walking. The DLA is divided into two parts: a care component for help with personal care needs which is paid at three different levels and a mobility component to help with walking difficulties paid at two levels.

Once again the requirements can be complicated and people should be encouraged to apply and, if unsuccessful, should be encouraged to appeal as there is quite a high success rate following the appeal procedure. The DLA acts as a gateway to certain other types of help including various disability premiums paid on top of other allowances and, for example, provides access to the Independent Living Fund. The old Attendance Allowance is still paid for people who are over 65 years old who are severely disabled and need help with personal care or supervision.

Providing care

An Invalid Care Allowance is a benefit for people under 65 who spend at least 35 hours a week caring for a severely disabled person. This was a useful and welcome piece of legislation that at last recognized the role of the informal carer.

Other benefits and grants

Other sources of help are available. The Independent Living Fund, for example, supplements funds available from the local authority and funds more expensive care packages for severely disabled people living at home. Social services departments are also allowed to make direct payments to individuals under the Community Care Direct Payments Bill 1996 so that individuals can buy in their own care rather than have it provided for them. Table 16.4

provides a very brief benefit checklist. Once again it should be emphasized that this table is over simplistic and proper advice is required from appropriate experts.

Disability increases costs and tends to reduce income and thus is a potential cause of poverty. This additional handicap can be ameliorated, at least to some extent, by taking full advantage of the range of social security and other payments applicable to disabled people and their carers.

Legal problems

Some people with disabilities have the right to legal redress. These individuals will usually have a disability as a result of personal injury caused by another party either directly or as a result of negligence or as a failure of duty of care. If there is any suggestion of the disability being caused by a third party legal advice is advisable as soon as possible. Even if the third party is unidentified, such as after a hit and run accident or by criminal injury, some compensation is still possible through the Motor Insurers Bureau or the Criminal Injuries Compensation Board. A total of 66 different diseases have been described as risks of particular occupations and can receive compensation. Support is also available through the War Disablement Pension or by a payment for those disabled by vaccine damage. There are lawyers who specialize in personal injury or medical negligence and it is important to obtain expert advice. A list of interested lawyers can be obtained from the Association of Personal Injury Lawyers (see Further Reading).

The legal process can be long, tedious, and complex but for some individuals can eventually provide access to sufficient funds to compensate for 'pain, suffering, and loss of amenity', provide for future care, equipment, and housing requirements, and compensate for lost earnings. The rehabilitation team should also remember that in certain circumstances the court can make a transitional payment in advance of a final settlement which may provide for a particular piece of equipment, housing

Table 16.4 Summary of current UK benefits system

Situation	Benefit available
Incapable of work: previously employed	Statutory Sick Pay/Incapacity Benefit
Incapable of work: insufficient NI contributions	Severe Disablement Allowance
Incapable of work: insufficient to live on	Income Support
Unemployed	Job Seekers Allowance/Income Support
Incapable of work	Job Seekers Allowance/Income Support
Working at least 16 hours a week	Disability Working Allowance
Injured or contracted disease at work	Industrial Injuries Disablement Benefit/ Reduced Earnings Allowance
Vaccine damage	Vaccine Damage Payment
Injury due to violent crime	Criminal Injuries Compensation
War disablement	War Disablement Pension/War Widows Pension
Retirement	Retirement Pension/Income Support
Help with personal care	Disability Living Allowance Care Component/Attendance Allowance/ Independent Living Funds
Problems with walking	Disability Living Allowance Mobility Component/Motability Scheme/Road Tax Exemption/Orange Badge Scheme
Practical help at home	Care services (home-help, meals-on-wheels) from social services and/or NHS
Help with NHS glasses, hospital fares	Health Benefits
Housing problems. renovation or other housing grants	Housing Benefit, Council Tax Benefit
Caring—for at least 35 hours a week	Invalid Care Allowance
Disabled children	Child Benefit/Guardian's Allowance/One Parent Benefit/Family Credit/ Disability Allowance/Family Fund/Health Benefits
Insufficient income	Income Support/Job Seekers Allowance/ Family Credit/Disability Working Allowance/Social Fund Community Care Grant/Budgeting Loan/Crisis Loan
Other	Other benefits from other government departments such as Department of Employment or local authority (e.g. leisure pass, bus pass) or private sector (e.g. rail passes)

adaptations, or even pay for some aspects of rehabilitation and care support staff. Eventual payment can now be considerable and investment advice may be required or payment can be staggered through a structured settlement. This is a complex and expert field and the rehabilitation team should have access to advice and help from a local interested and expert solicitor.

Carers

Around 90 per cent of care provided to disabled people at home is given by informal carers, such as partners or parents. People with severe disabilities can place major demands upon their main carer in terms of time, physical requirements, and psychological stress.

The first task for the rehabilitation team is to identify the potential carer or carers network. This is not always obvious. Occasionally apparently obvious carers are unwilling to change their lifestyle. The author remembers a long-standing partner of a head injured man who was widely assumed to be in a position to take on the caring role. However, it became clear that their relationship had been one that enabled them both to lead very independent lives and she was unwilling to change her lifestyle to accommodate caring for her long-standing partner. Such decisions should be respected and not readily criticized. Sometimes relationships are not all that they seem. For example, the parents of a severely disabled head injured young man wished to take him home as his residual disability made him heavily dependent upon others. It transpired that he had had a very unhappy and abused childhood and his girlfriend considered that the last place he would want to be was living back in the parental home. After some acrimony with his parents she eventually assumed the caring role herself. The pre-existing nature of the relationship should also be explored. Some relationships were difficult prior to any acquired disability and separation or divorce may have been pending. Guilt or obligation or pressure from the rehabilitation staff can lead a partner to assume a caring role which is unlikely to succeed if the relationship was poor beforehand. It is better to identify difficulties prior to discharge home. Particular caution should be exercised if a child is to look after a parent in any way. The parent/child role reversal involved in such situations will need careful exploration, is usually undesirable and may cause potential long-term psychological problems for the child.

Even if the main carer is entirely capable and willing caring is a stressful occupation. The carer will often require as much practical help at home as possible, particularly for more mundane housework or for very personal tasks that are more appropriately done by professionals. Psychological stress and anxiety should be recognized before major relationship problems occur. Depression is also common amongst carers. The carers are in just as much need of psychological support as well as information, advice, and counselling as the disabled person. Respite care would normally be part of a package for a severely disabled person. This can take many forms. Respite for a few hours a day, even intermittently, to enable the carer to get out alone, perhaps just for a shopping trip. Respite provided within the home to enable the carer a longer break away from home is also important although such facilities are few and far between. The classic respite break involves the disabled person being admitted to a residential or nursing home or hospital which may be less than desirable for the disabled person but essential for the carer and indeed may be a factor that allows long-term care in the community to continue. If there are local carer support groups these should be made known. Finally, rehabilitation teams should be able to explore the wider social network of the individual and encourage friends and relatives to be involved as appropriate, even on a very occasional basis, to allow a break for the main carer and immediate family.

Conclusions

This chapter has only briefly covered the whole range of issues pertinent to handicap. The rehabilitation team and rehabilitation physician may not be the best experts to advise on many of these issues but must have a grasp of the system and local knowledge in order to point the disabled person and their family in the right direction and reduce as far as possible the increased social problems that come with disability.

Further reading

Education and further education

Cole, T. (1986). *Residential special education: living and learning in a special school*. Open University Press, Milton Keynes.

Corlett, S. and Cooper, D. (1992). *Students with disabilities and higher education*. National Bureau for Students with Disabilities, London.

SKILL (1991). *A guideto higher education for people with disabilities (Part 1: Making your application; Part 2: A guide to Universities; Part 3: A guide to polytechnics, institutes and colleges of higher education)*. National Bureau for Students with Disabilities, London.

Warnock Report (1978). *Special education needs*. HMSO, London.

School leaver

Aung, T. S., Boughey, A. M., and Ward, A. B. (1994). The study of the North Staffordshire Young Adult Service for Physically Disabled School Leavers and Young Adults. *Clinical Rehabilitation*, **8**, 147–53.

Beardshaw, V. (1988). *The hidden 3,000, joint study of services for physically handicapped people in Gloucester*, vols 1–3. Social Services Department, Gloucestershire County Council.

Handoff, D. and Chigien, E. (1991). Developing community-based services for youth with disabilities. *Paediatrician*, **18**, 157–62

Prince of Wales Advisory Group on Disability (1985). *Living options*. Prince of Wales Advisory Group on Disability, London.

Ward, A. B. and Chamberlain, M. A. (1977). Enabling the young disabled adult. In: Goodwill, C. J., Chamberlain, M. A., and Evans, C. D. (ed.) *Rehabilitation of the physically disabled adult*, 2nd edn. Stanley Thornes, Cheltenham.

Employment

The Disability Alliance (1997–8). *Disability rights handbook*, 22nd edn. Disability Alliance, London.

Cantrell, E. (1997). Work, occupation and disability. In: Wilson, B. A. and McLellan, D. L. (ed.) *Rehabilitation studies handbook*, pp. 115–42. Cambridge University Press, Cambridge.

RADAR (1996). *Self-employment—a positive option—a guide for disabled people*. RADAR, London.

Further information on current services is offered by the Employment Service available from local office

Housing and home adaptations

Goldsmith, S. (1984). *Designing for the disabled*. RIBA Publications, London.

Miller, E. J. and Gwynne, G. V. (1972). *A life apart: a pilot study of residential institutions for the physically handicapped and the young chronic sick.* Tavistock Publications, London. (A classic study of life for young disabled people in institutions.)

Spencely, H. (1997). Housing issues. In: Barnes, M. P., Braithwaite, B., and Ward, A. B. (ed.) *Medical aspects of personal injury litigation*, pp.387–406. Blackwell Science, Oxford.

Leisure Interests

RADAR (1994). *Country parks*. RADAR, London.

RADAR (1997). *Holidays in the British Isles*. RADAR, London.

Thompson, N. (1984). *Sports and recreation—provision for the disabled.* Butterworths, London (published for the Disabled Living Foundation).

Walsh, A. (1991). *Nothing ventured—disabled people travel the world. A Rough Guide special.* Harrap Columbus, London.

Finance and benefits

Disability Alliance (1997). *Disability rights handbook*, 22nd edn. Disability Alliance, London.

Legal problems

Barnes, M. P., Braithwaite, B., and Ward, A. B. (1997). *Medical aspects of personal injury litigation*. Blackwell Science, Oxford.

Section E

....

Specific disabilities

17

....

Multiple sclerosis

Multiple sclerosis is an important cause of severe physical disability, particularly amongst young adults. The prevalence of the disease combined with the progressive and changing nature and complexity of the resulting disability makes multiple sclerosis one of the major challenges to the neurological rehabilitation team. The neurological literature contains much information regarding the aetiology, pathogenesis, and diagnostic aspects of multiple sclerosis compared with the paucity of the literature on the resulting disability and handicap. This chapter will concentrate on the management of disability but will mention some relevant points regarding epidemiology, natural history, and prognosis.

Epidemiology

There is a well known distinct geographical variation in the prevalence of the disease. There is a very strong trend for the prevalence to increase with increasing latitude both north and south of the equator. The trend is even noticeable in a country the size of the UK with lower prevalence rates reported towards the south of England compared with significantly higher rates in northern Scotland. The generally accepted prevalence rates in southern England are now around 120 per 100 000 population which has been reported to go up to about 250 per 100 000 population in northern Scotland. The incidence is around 2–6 per 100 000 population per annum. Thus, a typical group general practice with a population of 10 000 will have around 12 people with multiple sclerosis. Obviously in the early stages not all these individuals are disabled but overall about two-thirds of the multiple sclerosis population have a moderate or severe disability. People with multiple sclerosis are important consumers of health and social care in the UK. The mean age of onset of multiple sclerosis is around 30 with the burden of disability falling in the fourth and fifth decades of life. Thus, the disorder can cause significant handicap as it will often occur in an individual who is in work and with a young family.

Natural history

Life expectancy is overall slightly shortened in multiple sclerosis although there are many people with relatively benign disease who have quite normal life expectancy. At the other end of the spectrum there is a small proportion of people with rapidly progressive multiple sclerosis with death within a year or so of onset. The overall life expectancy has improved in recent years with better management of disability and handicap. Around 90 per cent of people with multiple sclerosis are still alive, albeit with disability, 40 years after onset.

There are a number of different patterns of multiple sclerosis. Around two-thirds of people will have a relapsing remitting course from the onset of disease with a further 15 per cent having a progressive course with superimposed acute episodes. Most of the remainder will have a chronically progressive course from onset. Eventually the great majority of people convert to a progressive phase, usually around 10–15 years from the onset of the disease. There is probably a small population of people, around 10 per cent of the total, who do not convert to progressive disease but continue to have a benign course with occasional relapses and remissions. The time interval between the onset of the disease and the start of the progressive phase is the best prognostic indicator. Those who become progressive within a short period are more likely to have aggressive disease.

It is difficult to predict the course of the disease with any accuracy. Generally cerebellar symptoms and signs carry a poor prognosis as does polysymptomatic onset. Monosymptomatic onset and visual and sensory symptoms in the early stages probably carry a better prognosis. The absence of pyramidal or cerebellar signs five years after onset is also a good indicator of benign disease. Increasing age of onset, particularly age of onset after 40, is a poor prognostic sign.

Diagnosis

A diagnosis of multiple sclerosis still largely rests on traditional clinical skills of history and examination in an attempt to identify clinical lesions in the central nervous system at two or more different anatomical sites that have occurred on at least two separate occasions. Clinical judgement can be backed up by evoked potential testing, examination of the spinal fluid, or more importantly by modern MRI neuroimaging. Overall it is now possible to give a good indication of the likelihood of multiple sclerosis at an early stage.

It is now generally accepted that individuals have a right to be told of the diagnosis or possible diagnosis as soon as possible. Most studies have shown that people wish to be told the diagnosis at the earliest possible stage. This phase of care is often poorly managed and a recent survey in Southampton showed that individuals still learn their diagnosis inappropriately and indeed 10 per cent had learnt by accident or by an incautious remark by a health-care professional. The majority of people still feel that insufficient detail is given about the disease at the time of diagnosis. It is important that information is given in an unhurried atmosphere, allowing the patient and family time to discuss and ask questions and preferably soon afterwards being given a second appointment when further questions are bound to have materialized. There is now useful literature written in lay terms produced by multiple sclerosis societies (see further reading) and books written by people who have multiple sclerosis. This literature is often very useful for the newly diagnosed individual and their family.

Precipitating and aggravating factors

In many cases a relapse in multiple sclerosis will occur without warning and without obvious reason. However, there are some risk factors that need to be borne in mind.

Pregnancy

There is a significant decrease in relapse rate during pregnancy, particularly during the third trimester. However, this is counterbalanced by a slightly increased relapse risk during the 3–6 months post partum. Overall the consensus is that pregnancy now has no long-term adverse effect on disability. The choice of whether to become pregnant clearly must lie with the couple involved but there is certainly no medical reason to advise against pregnancy in multiple sclerosis. There is no evidence that the contraceptive pill has a negative influence on the course of the disease.

Stress and life events

There is much speculation that stressful life events can influence the onset and later course of multiple sclerosis. There is no definitive proof that this is the case but there are now a large number of anecdotal reports in the literature that clearly show a relationship between a sudden stressful event and the onset of the disease or a relapse. Such events can include acute emotional shock, surgical operations, trauma, and systemic infections.

Rating scales

It is important to be able to record the extent of impairment, disability, and handicap in any individual with a long-term neurological condition. This will allow a more accurate indication to be made of prognosis and can facilitate the proper long-term planning of service delivery. It is now generally accepted that generic disability rating scales are probably more useful than scales relating to specific diseases. However, in multiple sclerosis there are very wildly used measures—the Kurtzke scales. Many centres now use the Kurtzke Expanded Disability Status Scale as a measure of impairment, the Kurtzke Incapacity Status Scale as a measure of disability, and the Environmental Status Scale as a measure of handicap. These scales are not entirely satisfactory but nevertheless have the advantage of being relatively quick to administer, are well known, and do provide a reasonably comprehensive assessment of impairment, disability, and handicap. Other appropriate scales to use in multiple sclerosis are discussed in Chapter 5.

Management of multiple sclerosis

Treatment to alter disease progression

For many years immunosuppression has been the mainstay of treatment in multiple sclerosis. Traditionally immunotherapy is initiated at times of acute relapse or occasionally at a very rapidly progressive phase of the disease. It would appear that the most effective treatment is intravenous methylprednisolone, usually administered at a dose of around 500 mg–1 g intravenously daily for three days. This is sometimes followed by a rapidly decreasing course of oral steroids. This treatment hastens recovery from the relapse but probably makes little long-term difference to the overall disease progression. Very occasionally there are individuals who seem to be steroid responsive in the longer term and appear to relapse when steroids are withdrawn or reduced. However, it is generally unwise to administer long-term steroids as in most people these will make no difference to the course of the disease and are associated with a significant range of troublesome side effects.

Other immunosuppressive agents have been used with modest effect including azathiopine and cyclophosphamide.

These drugs seem to stabilize or even improve the disease but only for a short period before reprogression.

More recently interferons have been introduced for the management of multiple sclerosis. Interferon beta-1a and interferon beta-1b (Avonex, Rebif, and Betaferon) are now available for prescription and appear to reduce relapse rate as well as reducing lesion load on serial MRI scanning. There is more recent evidence of some, albeit modest, reduction in disability in the long term associated with interferon therapy. Therapy is now usually restricted to those with frequent relapses. The treatment is relatively safe but there are disadvantages in that all currently available forms of interferon do require either subcutaneous or intramuscular injection several times a week. There is a range of other side effects including nausea, vomiting, headache, abdominal pain, and dizziness. Overall around 40 per cent of individuals do have some troublesome side effect on this treatment. A spin-off of the introduction of these therapies is the increasingly widespread employment of nurse practitioners with expertise in the field of multiple sclerosis. Many of these nurses were introduced by commercial organizations in order to administer interferon injection. However, their role has now expanded and there is an active MS Nurse Forum (sponsored by the Multiple Sclerosis (Research) Charitable Trust—see useful addresses). This organization is now developing a comprehensive training programme for nurses with skills and expertise in multiple sclerosis who should be an invaluable addition to the community support network.

A new drug which should be on the UK market in the near future is co-polymer 1 (Copaxone). This is shown to have a beneficial effect in patients with relapsing remitting disease causing a decrease in the number of relapses and also appears to have a modest, positive effect in terms of disability progression.

A variety of other treatments including cyclosporin, plasmapharesis, potassium channel blockers, monoclonal antibodies as well as various cytokines have now been used in small-scale human studies. Many of these compounds show some promise but none yet have proven value and most are still in the experimental stage.

Several of these therapies, including the interferon therapy currently on the market, are expensive. The cost of one individual on interferon treatment for one year is approximately £10 000 and purchasers of health care have difficult economic decisions to make. Ethical dilemmas will become increasingly common in this field. Is it, for example, of more overall benefit to employ one physiotherapist for a year than to treat two individuals with interferon therapy?

Diet

A few studies have demonstrated a modest reduction in relapse rate by use of a diet supplemented by both N6 and N3 polyunsaturated fatty acids, mainly eicosapentaenoic and docosahexaenoic acids. These compounds can be found in fish oils. Such diets are safe, and even if the benefit is modest most individuals report a positive psychological benefit from trying to do something themselves to ameliorate the disorder. Early studies in this field involved the use of evening primrose oil. This is still widely used by people with multiple sclerosis but has not been shown to have any clear physical benefit.

Management of major symptoms

The challenge for rehabilitation in multiple sclerosis is managing the complex interaction that lies behind the disability, often involving several different neuronal systems. There are few disorders that require so much active interdisciplinary cooperation from all members of the rehabilitation team. Table 17.1 summarizes symptoms, associated with and without difficulty in activities of daily living in a large sample of people with multiple sclerosis.

Mobility

Difficulty in walking is one of the most common symptoms in multiple sclerosis and the frequency approaches 100 per

Table 17.1 Symptoms in 656 people with multiple sclerosis (from Kraft *et al.* 1986)

Symptom present	No ADL (difficulty (%))	With ADL (difficulty (%))	Total (%)
Fatigue	21	56	77
Balance problems	24	50	74
Weakness or paralysis	18	45	63
Numbness, tingling, or other sensory disturbance	39	24	63
Bladder problems	25	34	59
Increased muscle tension (spasticity)	23	26	49
Bowel problems	19	20	39
Difficulty remembering	21	16	37
Depression	18	18	36
Pain	15	21	36
Laugh or cry easily (emotional lability)	24	8	32
Double or blurred vision, partial or complete blindness	14	16	30
Shaking (tremor)	14	13	27
Speech and/or communication difficulties	12	11	23
Difficulty solving problems	12	9	21

ADL=activities of daily living.

cent with time. Walking difficulties are often due to a combination of pyramidal weakness combined with spasticity but with major secondary effects from fatigue, disuse, pain, ataxia, sensory loss, and proprioceptive problems. Proper management of spasticity (see Chapter 6) and the prevention of contractures is vital. A structured exercise programme, planned and supervized by a physiotherapist, is also needed. Proper and timely use of mobility aids including canes, walkers or orthoses, and eventually wheelchairs is clearly part of ongoing physiotherapy support. Hydrotherapy is useful as a further aid to both increased activity and range of movement and additionally has an anti-spastic effect. When individuals are less active, passive stretching and range of movement exercises are still vital in order to maintain as much function as possible and prevent contractures.

Upper limb function

A combination of pyramidal weakness combined with spasticity, ataxia, and sensory disturbance can amount to significant arm disability. The occupational therapist and physiotherapist should be involved in the management of people with significant arm problems. Exercises to utilize activities of daily living to improve dexterity and coordination are important. There are a variety of simple aids that can make hand and arm tasks much simpler. In the UK there is a network of Disabled Living Centres and National Demonstration Centres where such equipment is displayed and appropriate advice can be given. Proper management of spasticity is once again important.

Cerebellar dysfunction

Unfortunately cerebellar involvement is common and difficult to treat. Occasionally there is modest benefit from treatment with isoniazid, choline, benzodiazepines, sodium valproate, or botulinum toxin intramuscular injections. However, most such treatment is unhelpful and individuals have to rely on adaptive equipment or simple orthotic devices such as weighted bands on the wrists, large handled implements, plate guards and velcro fastenings for buttons and shoelaces, electric toothbrushes, electric page turners, and a variety of other useful aids. Occasional severe intention tremor can be treated by cryothalamotomy.

Swallowing disorders

Significant swallowing disorders are uncommon until later stage disease. Bronchopneumonia is still the leading cause of death in multiple sclerosis and it is likely swallowing difficulties are under-recognized. Swallowing involves a

highly complex motor sequence and requires expert
evaluation by a speech and language therapist as well as
a dietician and radiographer. Videofluroscopy is essential
to make a proper study of dysphagic problems. The subject
is covered more fully in Chapter 9. If there are difficulties
with oral feeding it is better to move sooner rather than
later to feeding through a percutaneous endoscopic gastrostomy. However, ethical dilemmas may arise regarding
whether such active intervention is required at end stage
disease.

Communication problems

Dysphasia is unusual in multiple sclerosis. Most communication problems arise from cerebellar or spastic dysarthria. Referral to a speech and language therapist can be
useful in improving functional communication skills. If
such improvement is not possible then referral to a
communication aids centre, specializing in augmentative
communication devices, can produce a gratifying improvement in the quality of life.

Continence

Urinary problems are extremely common in multiple
sclerosis and are probably responsible for more handicap
than any other problem. The most common symptom is
urgency, reported in up to three-quarters of people with
multiple sclerosis at some stage of the disease. Urge incontinence occurs in around half of the population at some
point, as does frequency. Symptoms associated with
bladder hypoactivity (hesitancy, overflow incontinence,
use of abdominal pressure when voiding, and episodes of
retention) are less usual but still occur in about one-third
of individuals. The underlying pathophysiological problem is usually detrusor hyperreflexia often associated with
detrusor sphincter dyssynergia. A smaller proportion of
people have detrusor areflexia or hyporeflexia. The incidence of upper urinary tract involvement is fortunately
uncommon and should be preventable with adequate
urological follow-up. Urodynamic assessment is often

necessary. However, with symptoms of frequency, urgency and urge incontinence a trial of anticholinergic medication is probably justified prior to formal urodynamic assessment. A determination of residual volume is also necessary, preferably carried out by ultrasound. A residual volume greater than 100 ml is an indication for catheterization. It is best performed by intermittent catheterization either by the person with multiple sclerosis or a third party and is certainly preferable to a permanent indwelling catheter or suprapubic drainage. The reader is referred to Chapter 7 for more information on incontinence.

Bowel problems

Bowel difficulties in multiple sclerosis usually take the form of constipation or more rarely frequency and urgency. It is best to avoid medication if at all possible and more benefit is usually gained from attention to timing and amount of time spent in defecation as well as the maximal use being made of the gastrocolic reflex. Digital rectal stimulation or abdominal pressure are other useful mechanisms to promote defecation as well as a diet high in fibre and supplemented if needed by bulking agents, including an adequate water intake. Occasionally stool softeners such as sodium docusate can be helpful and only as a last resort should laxatives and enemas be applied.

Sexual function

Sexual problems are common in multiple sclerosis and under-recognized by health professionals. In women sexual difficulties often centre on fatigue and decreased sensation, libido, and orgasm whilst in men the main difficulty is centred on achieving and maintaining an erection combined with fatigue and decreased libido. Psychotherapy and psychosexual counselling should always be considered in combination with practical advice. Timing of intercourse with regard to fatigue, optimization of medication, reduced spasticity, correct advice on bladder management, and advice on positioning can all be helpful. Erectile dysfunction in the male can be helped by the use of prostaglandin E alprostadil (Caverject, Muse, and Viridal). These compounds are usually given by intra-cavernous injection. They have vaso-active properties which provide artificial erection through inhibition of alpha 1 adronergic activity and relaxation of the cavernosal smooth muscle. Recently Sildenafil (Viagra) has also been licensed for usage in the UK and is administered in tablet form. Sildenfail is a potent and selective inhibitor of the enzyme phosphodiesterase type 5 which prevents the degradation of cyclic GMP which in turn enhances the erectile response induced by sexual stimulation.

Problems with regard to sexual attitudes, sexual awareness, and self-image can often be improved by sensitive psychosexual counselling (see Chapter 8).

Pain and paroxysmal symptoms

Around one-third of people with multiple sclerosis have clinically significant pain at some point. This can be due to a variety of problems including musculo-skeletal pain from postural and gait abnormalities, pain from spasticity, or neuralgic pain as a direct result of the multiple sclerosis process. Often all three factors are operating and each factor will need treatment in its own right. Paroxysmal attacks often respond dramatically to carbamazepine therapy. Other paroxysmal symptoms can also occur in multiple sclerosis including paroxysmal dysarthria, ataxia, diplopia, and itch and all of these can be helped by carbamazepine.

Visual disturbance

Optic neuritis is one of the main presenting symptoms of multiple sclerosis and the treatment of choice is corticosteroid therapy. Other common problems including residual scotomas, diplopia, and oscillopsia all of which are rather difficult to treat. Occasionally symptomatic nystagmus can be helped with converging prisms or botulinum toxin therapy. Referral to a low-vision clinic can be helpful.

Fatigue

Fatigue is undoubtedly the commonest symptom in multiple sclerosis. It can have an overriding effect on the person's daily living activities and be the predominant reason for problems with employment and home life. Fatigue in multiple sclerosis can be related to depression which will need treatment in its own right but more commonly seems to be a direct result of the multiple sclerosis process, partly related to the high energy cost of walking but in some people apparently being caused independently of higher energy demands. Management depends on frequent rest periods during the day. Often more activities are possible in the morning than in the afternoon. A number of recent studies have shown a positive effect from amantidine therapy.

Cognitive dysfunction

Although impairment of intellectual function was recognized by early authors such as Charcot and l'Hermitte it is surprising that traditional teaching tends to underemphasize the importance of cognitive problems in multiple sclerosis. There is no doubt that cognitive impairment can be detected by neuropsychological testing even early in the course of the disease. Memory difficulties are common as are problems with information processing speed. It is important to recognize cognitive dysfunction in order to inform and reassure the person and family. Early referral to a neuropsychologist is important as coping strategies can be designed producing real functional benefit.

Emotional problems

Depression is common in multiple sclerosis, and various studies have shown that it occurs in up to 50 per cent of the population at some point. Clinical anxiety is a further problem, often compounded by lack of proper information. Unfortunately some physicians take a nihilistic view of depression and anxiety in multiple sclerosis—'Well they would be depressed wouldn't they'. This attitude is unhelpful and depression and anxiety need active treatment and intervention either by psychology, counselling, or psychiatric colleagues.

Many textbooks refer to euphoria being common in multiple sclerosis, although this is actually quite unusual. A few people seem to develop pathological laughing and crying which is usually effectively and quickly treated by a small dose of a tricyclic antidepressant.

Handicap

Problems in multiple sclerosis can often be unnecessarily compounded by lack of knowledge regarding local services and facilities that can reduce handicap. Health professionals should be acquainted with:
- local accessible leisure pursuits
- day centre provision
- respite care provision
- how to access local housing and housing adaptation systems
- welfare rights advice
- employment rehabilitation services
- carer support groups
- information and advice service
- contact address of local and national multiple sclerosis societies and other self-help groups.

A particular point to emphasize is the importance of employment rehabilitation. A study has indicated that 80 per cent of the economic loss to the national economy from people with multiple sclerosis is accounted for by lost earnings. The unemployment rate amongst the multiple sclerosis population is extremely high and in most studies exceeds 50 per cent. Proper advice and access to employment rehabilitation and retraining should be able to reduce this unnecessary burden.

Overall service delivery

The needs of the patients and families focus on the following:

1. Time—to discuss diagnosis and treatment as well as more personal cognitive and emotional difficulties. A counsellor attached to the multiple sclerosis team is a valuable asset.
2. Information—at the time of diagnosis and in the longer term to keep up to date with research and potential treatments.
3. Practical help—in terms of the provision of aids and equipment as well as access to personal help within the home.
4. Carers' needs—an equal need for access to information and counselling support as well as the need for access to respite facilities.

These needs are most readily provided within a health setting by a multidisciplinary team and a number of centres in the UK have now established a team dedicated to the needs of people with multiple sclerosis. The team often works in the community although access to hospital facilities is important as is access to other social service and voluntary facilities such as respite care, day centres, leisure interests, and employment expertise. It has now been shown that a dedicated community-based multiple sclerosis team produces real psychological and social benefit to the individual and reduces the risk of unnecessary physical complications. The person with multiple sclerosis and their families are better informed and better supported by such a system. The recent development of a network of nurse specialists in the field of multiple sclerosis is also a welcome addition to the overall community support network. The nurses should be invaluable and important members of community rehabilitation teams.

Conclusions

Multiple sclerosis is a common neurological disorder that produces a complex interaction of physical, psychological, social, and vocational problems. Access to an interdisciplinary rehabilitation team is vital in order to minimize disability and handicap and ensure that individuals and their families are given adequate information, explanation, and treatment wherever possible. Progressive neurological disease can produce an air of therapeutic nihilism but the rehabilitation team should be able to rise to the challenge and in all individuals promote improvement in the quality of life.

Reference

Kraft, G. H., Freal, J. E. and Coryll, J. K. (1986). Disability, disease duration and rehabilitation service needs in multiple sclerosis: patient perspectives. *Archives of Physical Medicine and Rehabilitation*, **67**, 164–78.

Further reading

Barnes, M. P. (1993). Multiple sclerosis. In: Greenwood, R., Barnes, M. P., McMillan, T. M., and Ward, C. D. (ed.) *Neurological rehabilitation*, pp.485–505. Churchill Livingstone, London.

Burnfield, A. (1996). *Multiple sclerosis: a personal exploration*. Souvenir Press, London.

Graham, J. (1987). *Multiple sclerosis: a self-help guide to its management*. Harper Collins, London.

Kraft, G. H. and Catanzano, M. (1996). *Living with MS: a wellness approach*. Demos Vermande, New York.

Raine, C. S., McFarland, H. F. and Tourtellotte, W. W. (ed.) (1997). *Multiple sclerosis—clinical and pathogenetic basis*, (2nd edn). Chapman and Hall, London.

Robinson, I. (1988). *Multiple sclerosis: experience of illness*. Routledge, London.

Useful addresses

Multiple Sclerosis (Research) Charitable Trust
Spirella Building
Bridge Road
Letchworth
Herts SG6 4ET, UK
Tel: 01462 675613

(The MSRCT produces a useful literature pack for people with
multiple sclerosis and health professionals.)

MS Society of Great Britain
25 Effie Road
Fulham
London SW6 1EE, UK
Tel: 0171 736 6267

18

....

Stroke

The management and rehabilitation of patients who have suffered a stroke is a major part of the work of clinicians in rehabilitation medicine and forms a significant proportion of the workload of rehabilitation units. Recent developments in stroke care have shown that dedicated services can not only save lives, but can optimize the potential for recovery and for coping with any subsequent disability. As a result, many purchasers and providers of health services are involved in the planning of more specialized services for hospital and community based care, and rehabilitation physicians have a significant role in ensuring that patients have equitable access to rehabilitation in both environments.

The term stroke is often referred to as a cerebrovascular accident, but stroke is better in rehabilitation settings. There are many causes, but the three most important in rehabilitation are those due to intracerebral haemorrhage, cerebral infarction, and subarachnoid haemorrhage. It is important to distinguish these three, not only because of the differing factors in primary and secondary prevention, but also because of some differing rehabilitative needs. In particular, and in contrast to cerebral infarction and cerebral haemorrhage, subarachnoid haemorrhage often presents as a more global disability, producing significant cognitive as well as physical problems and, in many cases, its rehabilitation is similar to that required for traumatic brain injury.

....

People have started to use the term 'brain attack', to compare the urgency of dealing with strokes with that of heart attack. This may be somewhat dramatic, but does signify that early intervention does bring benefits, both in terms of mortality and morbidity.

This chapter will look mainly at the important aspects in the rehabilitation of stroke patients, and aims to give the reader an insight into some of the issues affecting the stroke sufferer and his/her family/carers.

Epidemiology

Stroke is common; the annual incidence of first strokes is 200 per 100 000 population. A proportion of these will have a transient cerebral ischaemic attack with symptoms lasting for not more than 24 hours, but of those surviving an established stroke, about a half will be left disabled. The prevalence is around 550 per 100 000 of whom 300 will have a significant disability. In the average health district, there will therefore be about 1400 new strokes, of whom about half will be admitted to hospital. Two-thirds of these will occur in people over the age of 65 years. About 30 per cent of people with completed strokes die within a month, mainly from myocardial infarction, bronchopneumonia, and further stroke. The prevalence of disability due to stroke is about 400 people in every average health district, i.e. 250 000 people. The most common resultant disability is weakness but communication problems are also significant. About 15 to 20 per cent of stroke sufferers are left with a significant dysphasia and a further 10 per cent are documented as having a cognitive deficit (i.e. a problem with memory, perception, intellect, and other higher cerebral functioning). It has to be said that there is a significant unknown number of people with undetected cognitive disturbance.

Classification and diagnosis

The clinical diagnosis of a stroke is quite easy and the essential feature is the onset of neurological loss over a short period of time. The majority occur over a period of under an hour, although some may take a day or more to evolve. The classification shown below is adopted by the Royal College of Physicians, and is useful in clinical situations:

1. Transient cerebral ischaemic attack. Rapid onset of neurological symptoms under an hour, with full resolution within 24 hours.
2. Subarachnoid haemorrhage. Bleeding from intracranial vessels. This often arises from a 'berry' aneurysm situated in the intracerebral circulation and blood in the subarachnoid space often stimulates intense vaso-constriction, producing more widespread and diffuse symptoms than are seen in intracerebral haemorrhage or infarction.
3. Intracerebral haemorrhage. Sudden onset producing rapid neurological impairment, often associated with loss of consciousness.
4. Cerebral infarction. Neuronal loss in the brain due to localized impairment of cerebral circulation, resulting from either a cerebral embolus, or more commonly, from platelet micro-emboli due to progressive arteriosclerosis. The main associations are arterio-sclerotic cerebro-vascular disease and diabetes.

The impairments resulting from stroke depend on the location of the lesion. Figure 18.1 shows important features in the cerebral circulation. The circle of Willis forms a connecting ring between the carotid and vertebro-basilar trees and the middle cerebral artery can be seen arising from the circle in close association with the internal carotid artery which provides the main input of blood. Middle cerebral artery lesions are the most common in stroke, and classically affect the function of the internal capsule through which pass tightly packed motor and sensory nerve fibres to and from the contralateral side of the body. Also in close association is the optic radiation, passing back from the optic chiasma through the parietal lobe to the occipital cortex and interference of this will produce a contra-lateral homonymous hemianopia. Figures 18.2(a) and (b) show the deficits due to an interruption of the visual pathway.

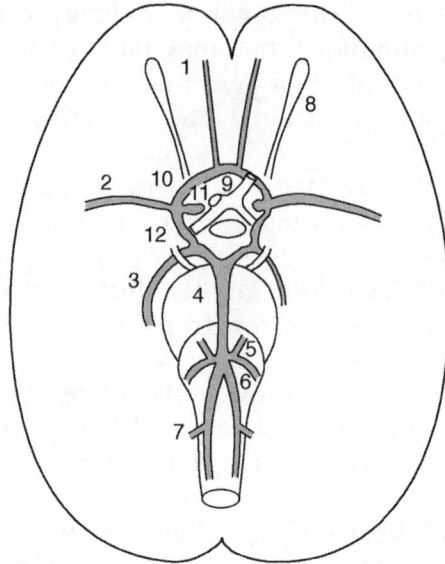

1. Anterior cerebral artery
2. Middle cerebral artery
3. Posterior cerebral artery
4. Basilar artery
5. Anterior inferior cerebellar artery
6. Vertebral artery

7. Posterior inferior cerebellar artery
8. Olfactory bulb
9. Optic Chiasma
10. Anterior communicating artery
11. Internal carotid artery
12. Posterior communicating artery

Fig. 18.1 Circle of Willis.

The term lacunar infarct is worth more detailed description. These are often multiple and result from occlusion of small arteries of 50–150 mm in diameter. They are associated with hypertension and arteriosclerosis and give rise to multiple deep small cavities, known as lacunae. They produce four specific syndromes which are as follows:

1. Hemiparesis with ataxia affecting the leg more than the arm (from an infarct in the internal capsule).
2. Pure motor hemiplegia (from an infarct in the pons or internal capsule).
3. Dysarthric-clumsy hand syndrome (pons)—dysarthria, slight dysphagia, central facial weakness, deviation of tongue to affected side, and clumsiness and ataxia in ipsilateral hand to side of lesion.

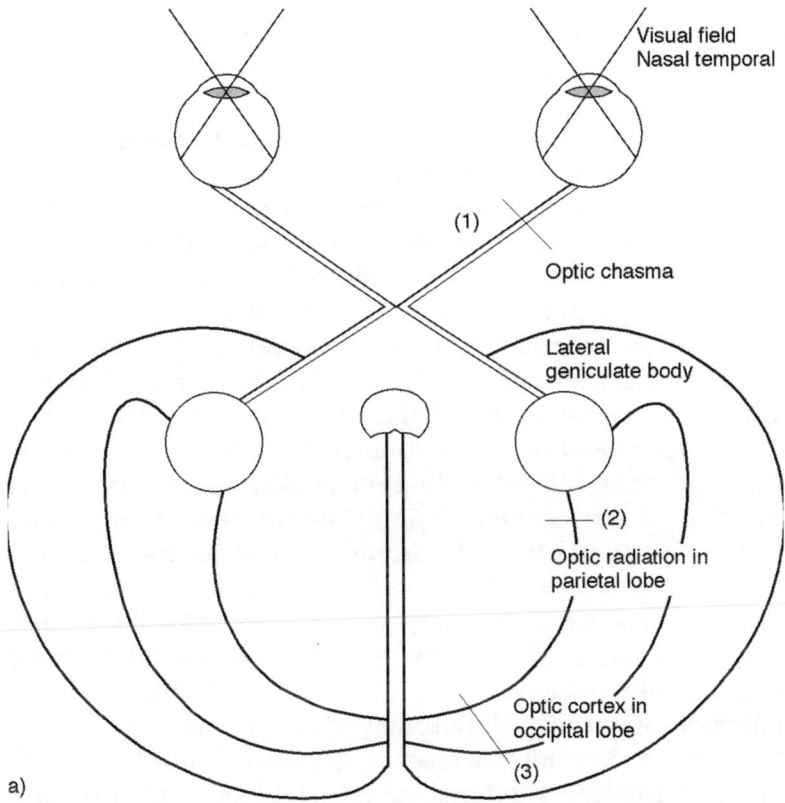

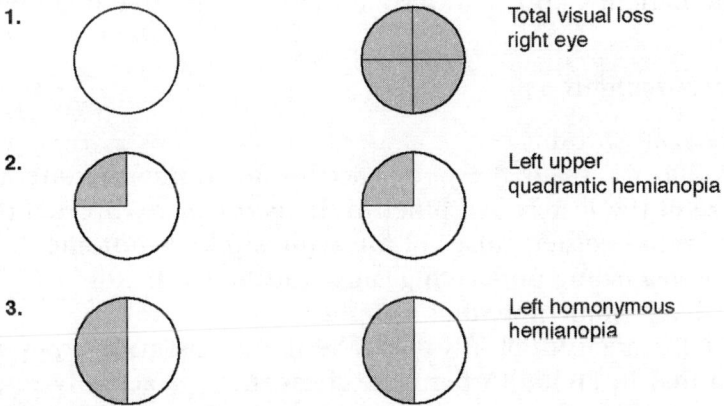

Fig. 18.2 (a) Visual pathways showing effects of lesions in optic nerve (1) and optic radiation (2) and (3); (b) Deficits due to interruption of visual pathway.

....

4. Pure sensory stroke with unilateral sensory loss for all
   modalities of sensation (posterolateral thalamic nucleus
   infarct).

More rare syndromes, such as lateral medullary syndromes,
can be found in more detail in a neurology text.

A lot of work has been carried out over recent years to
attempt to map the brain and we now have a better knowledge of the areas of the brain responsible for certain
activities. Dominance of one side of the brain is particularly
important in determining function, as well as in determining
whether the individual will become left or right-handed.
Table 18.1 shows some of the expected problems to arise
from impairment of the cerebral circulation, and highlights
the importance in rehabilitation of determining the exact
location of the cerebral lesion. For instance, frontal lobe
lesions, particularly at the fronto-parietal junction, have a
profound effect on the drive of the individual. Depression
may be suspected, but anti-depressants may have little
beneficial effect. Depression is very common after stroke
and usually responds well to medication, but, in these
patients, direct stimulation may give a better response, as
the problem lies not in a reactive depression, but in a loss of
drive or inertia. Similarly, mood problems and difficulty
with memory can be expected in *dominant* temporal lobe
lesions, and obviously, this will have a profound effect on
the patient's ability to respond to rehabilitative treatment.

Investigations

The completed stroke
Urgent CT scans are performed to determine the site and
size of the lesion. All other investigations are directed to:
• exclude other causes of the acute stroke syndrome
• reveal some underlying cause for the stroke, or
• detect some potential complication of a stroke.

CT scans cannot always make the diagnosis, as they are
normal in about 15 per cent of cases. They actually rarely
change the management of the patient, but are essential in
four specific situations:
1. To exclude cerebral haemorrhage when anti-coagulant
   or anti-platelet treatment is being considered.

Table 18.1 Localizing features of brain disease

Site	Impairments/deficits
Frontal lobe	Behavioural abnormalities, Planning/anticipatory difficulties. Inertia and decreased initiative
Parietal lobe	Spatial disorientation. Apraxia. Agnosia. Sensory inattention. Receptive dysphasia*. Homonymous hemianopia[†]
Pre-central gyrus (within parietal lobe)	Localized weakness/monoplegia. Expressive dysphasia
Post central gyrus	Localized sensory loss
Temporal lobe	Memory. Hallucination (auditory and visual). Decreased concentration/attention. Receptive dysphasia . Quadratic hemianopia
Occipital lobe	Hemianopia
Base of brain	Hemiplegia and hemi-anaesthesia. Spasticity++cranial nerve deficits
Brain stem	Ataxia. Cranial nerve problems, particularly dysarthria and diplopia. Spasticity+++. Diffuse (as found in SAH). Decreased information processing. Decreased IQ. Cognitive problems

* Non-dominant hemisphere.
[†] Dominant hemisphere.
SAH: subarachnoid haemorrhage.

2. When there is a suspicion that a patient has an intra-cranial mass due to tumour, subdural haematoma, or abscess.
3. When intracranial hypertension is suspected, particularly if the patient's level of consciousness is dropping and surgical intervention is being considered.
4. When the patient's course is atypical and the diagnosis is in doubt.

Table 18.2 gives an outline of the typical investigations. In comparison to stroke, all other causes are uncommon, if not rare. However, many require specific treatment.

Tumours and subdural haematomas require surgical advice; post-epileptic paresis, non-specific alterations in consciousness, and biochemical abnormalities require investigation although they only rarely cause a stroke. As myocardial disease is the commonest cause of death following stroke, a thorough examination and assessment of the heart is important. Atrial fibrillation should be treated with anti-coagulants, in the absence of cerebral haemorrhage. Atrial fibrillation is found as commonly in cerebral haemorrhage as it is in infarction, and just because it is found, does not mean it is the cause of the stroke. However, the risk is higher, particularly if patients are moving in and out of sinus rhythm.

Table 18.2   Investigations

FBC, ESR, clotting screen*
Biochemical screen, HbA$_1$C, Thyroid function tests
Cholesterol subsets, triglyceride
ECG
Echocardiogram*
EEG*
CT scan
Doppler scan*

* if clinically indicated

Transient ischaemic attacks (TIAs)

TIAs require full investigation, as it is important to prevent completed strokes. Successful intervention of a TIA has a beneficial effect on outcome, and certainly this 'warning' should not go unheeded. Reducing the risk factors for stroke is important and centres on the treatment of hypertension, the prevention of smoking, the control of diabetes, and the detection and treatment of other rarer abnormalities, such as anaemia, polycythaemia etc. However, enthusiastic searching for an occult cause is not particularly valuable and correction of the major associations is a more important activity.

Any patient with a transient ischaemic attack should be referred for specialist investigation and neurological services are becoming organized to provide the necessary facilities. Arrhythmias are straightforward to detect and should be treated appropriately. The major cause of transient ischaemic attacks is from arteriosclerosis (whether or not this is compounded by hypertensive changes or by diabetes), but occasionally significant carotid artery occlusion is treatable by endarterectomy, thus decreasing the risk of further stroke. Auscultating over the neck for carotid bruits is therefore valuable and simple to perform. No specific focal lesion is found in the majority of TIAs and anti-thrombotic treatment with aspirin should be started. In contraindicated patients, dipyridamole can be used as an alternative and evidence is growing to support the benefits of combining these two drugs for most patients. Reduction of risk factors by health education is vital for the prevention of a completed stroke, i.e. cessation of smoking, weight reduction in obese people, lipid reduction, optimal control of diabetes, and increasing physical activity.

Rehabilitation of the completed stroke patient

The development of a stroke is particularly frightening for both the patient and his/her family. It must be met with the demonstration of knowledge and skills in dealing with the condition in order to give patients and their families the confidence that an appropriate response is being made.

Depending on local factors, a proportion of patients will be managed at home following their stroke. They too require investigation and the general practitioner may call upon the advice of specialist help. However, the majority of significantly disabled patients are admitted to hospital and this is the most common route to specialist rehabilitation. This book will not discuss controversial management of the impairment, such as thrombolysis, but will concentrate on the assessment and management of disabled people following a completed stroke. The chapter therefore focuses on the medical assessment of patients, which has an impact in rehabilitation terms and gives an informed opinion on the likely outcome. Thereafter, issues on the support and follow-up of stroke patients will be mentioned.

Assessment of a stroke patient

A comprehensive history (which may have to be provided by a relative in patients with communication or cognitive problems) and examination are important. Neither may have been carried out in sufficient detail during the acute admission, but the greater time allowed in a rehabilitation environment makes this a thoroughly worthwhile activity. The history should now be redirected away from the patho-logical diagnosis (i.e. the stroke) towards identification of the impairments, disabilities, and handicaps. The bedside assessment should include detailed documentation of the physical and nutritional status of the patient, the motor and sensory deficit (including in particular, the presence of visual field defects) the presence of incontinence, tissue viability problems, spasticity, dysphagia (due to poor bulbar function), communication difficulties, and cognitive deficits. The patient's domestic situation and social history are of vital importance for rehabilitation and the health of carers and their ability to carry out care functions requires knowledge early on following the stroke. Pre-existing and comorbid disease may act as a barrier to successful progress in the rehabilitation process and a thorough understanding of its impact on the disability and lifestyle of the patient is valuable. There is no such thing as a 'simple stroke', since neither the disabilities nor the patient's circumstances are ever straightforward. Each patient needs individual consideration within a standard plan for assessment, which should include their mood and motivation. Mood changes, especially in younger patients after a stroke should not be considered particularly abnormal, but where they are likely to interfere with the rehabilitation process and with the patient's ability to make functional gains, they require treatment. Medication is now safe and widely available and the combination of this and good education is widely employed. Patients with communication disorders are particularly likely to become depressed and the sheer frustration of being unable to communicate their feelings to either their family or professionals may compound the situation further. Those with cognitive problems may be unable to benefit from rehabilitation because they simply cannot carry out the required tasks. Some patients are just not motivated for one reason or another to achieve the potential that others may think is possible and family members may not also be able to cope with the burden of care resulting in a significant failure of patients' marriages when this burden becomes clear. It is thus important to take all these aspects into consideration, for successful rehabilitation depends on identifying what the patients and carers want (and these may be different from each other) and what the professional team can deliver in order to produce realistic, achievable, and desired goals.

Sensory changes are important to elicit. They often present as abnormal sensation rather than outright numbness. Dysaesthesia and paraesthesiae can be very distressing and are referred to as cortical dysaesthesia/paraesthesia. Treatment with anti-convulsants, particularly Carbamazepine, can help some patients, but more aggressive treatment may be necessary.

So what are the expected deficits from our knowledge of brain mapping? An infarct in the cortex for instance, may give rise to a fairly limited motor or sensory loss, whereas one at the base of the brain, where nerve fibres are tightly packed, is likely to have a more devastating effect, which is likely to last for longer. However, many patients have a combination of both, for middle cerebral artery territory strokes are the most frequent and take the largest proportion of the circulation from the internal carotid artery and the Circle of Willis.

Although CT scanning is important, the main issues in predicting outcome are clinically based. Because 40 per cent of patients die within the first month, predictors of early mortality have been identified and are listed below:

- Capillary abnormalities
- Gaze paresis
- Abnormal respiratory pattern
- Bilateral extensor plantar responses.

In addition, the persistence of hypertension and significant cardiac disease are also predictors of a poor prognosis, even if the patient survives the first month.

Prognostic scores have been developed, which, if present four weeks after the stroke, predict a poor outcome at 15 weeks. In addition, low scores in the Barthel Scale of activities of daily living (ADL) at one month predict functional dependence at six months. Both pre-existing incontinence and early post-stroke incontinence are universally bad prognostic indicators, no matter what the underlying condition. The following are poor prognostic signs at one week:

- MRC grade 0 power in upper limb
- Unable to locate affected thumb with eyes closed
- Cannot maintain sitting balance
- Incontinence
- Loss of consciousness at onset.

It is somewhat easier to identify those patients who are going to do well after a stroke. It is, however, more difficult to determine those who will require more specialized help than those who would return to independence in any case. Early return of hand movement and shoulder protraction bode well for prehensile function and activities of daily living. Youth, and a motivation to achieve realistic targets, are important, and essentially the reverse of those features listed above, lead to less severe disability. Social circumstances (socio-economic class, wealth, home ownership, and a good supportive family) can affect the chance of a patient living at home, but they are not, somewhat strangely, indicators *per se* of a good prognosis in terms of independent living. Good cognition and communication and the ability to move the thumb and the foot are better. The combination of spontaneous recovery and good early rehabilitation can achieve much, but there are some factors, which, if they persist, will have an implication on the outcome, namely: inability to walk, loss of arm function, loss of postural control, hemianopia, proprioceptive sensory loss, spatial neglect, and impaired cognition.

Similarly, many people with strokes have concomitant problems, which act as rate-limiting barriers to successful rehabilitation:

1 Pre-existing physical disability—joint or cardiopulmonary disease.
2. Multiple pathology, e.g. loss of limb.
3. Sensory handicap.
4. Complications of disabling disease—incontinence, pressure sores, and impairment of intellect, memory, perception, communication, mood.

In some people, the stroke may appear as one of the final events of their life and heralds a multiorgan failure state.

Special points in assessment

History taking and examination are important, not only for identifying prognostic factors, but for providing medical input into the rehabilitation process.

Motor function

Measurement of upper limb power is often of little value in stroke and recording the limb function usually gives more useful information. Dexterity and shoulder function should be determined, as well as the ability to initiate movements, particularly in the arm. Grip, pinch grip, and the ability to raise the hand to the mouth or occiput, have implications on personal function, particularly in respect of feeding and grooming oneself. Where walking is possible, simple tests, such as measuring the walking speed with a 10 m walking time, gives valuable information, which can be performed repeatedly to measure progress. If muscle power is measured, comparison against the opposite is feasible, or, if that is not possible (such as in the loss of limb), then comparison can be made against the examiner's own power. The ability to make controlled movements in a functional way is important to document. One should also carry out an objective measurement of spasticity. The modified Ashworth Scale has not been validated in stroke, but is clinically valuable.

Sitting posture must be controlled before standing and walking. Ataxia compromises sitting posture and training is required so that these patients can cope with their in-coordination rather than try to reduce it. It is also important to record hand dominance in order to predict the potential deficits, such as dysphasia, dyspraxia, spatial attention, and non-verbal communication skills.

Swallowing

The incidence of dysphagia following stroke is about 10 per cent, although it is thought that many patients have unrecognized problems. A good bedside test is to measure the time taken to drink 150 ml of water. If there is any choking, the test should be aborted immediately and suction should always be at hand to deal with any problems. People with normal swallowing functions can usually manage this quantity of fluid within 10 to 12 s. If dysphagia is found, referral to a speech and language therapist is indicated to utilize their specialized skills.

Sensation

Altered sensation is associated with a less favourable outcome, as the lack of feedback gives rise not only to poor limb positioning and therefore spasticity, but also to an inability to undertake mobility and dexterity training. Proprioceptive loss has a profound adverse effect on the achievement of independence and measures to stimulate this can be affected by good positioning by nursing staff and constant reminding for visual confirmation of the limb's position. Sensory inattention and perceptual loss are often considered as part of the sensory deficit, but in this context, they will be discussed under cognitive impairment.

Vision

Visual field loss is disabling, especially in the context of hemiplegia or cognitive loss. Confrontation testing is performed by asking the patient to point to the examiner's moving fingers with the unaffected hand. Visual inattention is assessed by bilateral simultaneous confrontation and visual neglect and agnosia by making drawings and facial recognition respectively. Both hemianopia and visual inattention have an implication, both for the ability of the patient to utilize a powered wheelchair, or to drive a car. Some patients have a partial loss such as a quadrantic loss and it is advisable that formal visual field test by perimetry is undertaken when it is suspected.

Communication

Verbal communication (articulation, language, voice, and fluency) and non-verbal communication require detailed assessment. The role of the nursing staff cannot be underestimated in providing the right conditions to initiate communication and become an information resource. Obviously, a speech and language therapist will be required, particularly for retraining in dysarthria (articulation problems) and in the rehabilitation of language problems. Articulation, voice, and fluency are often frequently impaired by faulty voice control and usually improve. They are much more common in non-dominant hemisphere strokes. Language disorders (aphasia) on the other hand (comprehension, expression, spelling, and writing) are one of the most disabling features of a stroke and various studies suggest that between 21 and 24 per cent of stroke patients admitted to hospital have a language disorder. Ten to 18 per cent of long-term survivors are significantly affected. It is probably advisable to leave detailed assessment to the speech and language therapist, as one of the strategies in dysphasia is to set up a consistent communication method which the patient can understand.

Inexpert attempts may result firstly in confusion and secondly distress to the patient and relatives. It is most important to identify whether the patient has true preservation of comprehension, as opportunities for participation in rehabilitation will be that much greater. In these patients, communication aids are possible and these may range from simple writing pads to letter boards and more sophisticated aids, which can be linked with environmental control systems. Comprehension (the ability to understand the spoken word) is sometimes difficult to assess and many relatives will say that the patient can understand more then the professionals realize. It is therefore important to have an objective reproducible assessment. Complex ideational comprehension can be tested by using a simple plan as below in which one point is scored for each correct answer:

'Mr. Jones had to go to London. He decided to take the train and his wife drove him to the station, but on the way they had a flat tyre. The wheel was changed and they arrived at the station just in time for him to catch the train.'

Questions:
1. Did Mr. Jones catch the train?
2. Did he get to the station on time?
3. Did the train have a flat tyre?
4. Was Mr. Jones going to London?
5. Was he on his way home from London?

Higher cerebral functions

Cognitive disorders (attention, memory, thinking, problem-solving, judgement, language, and number), perceptional disorders (visuospatial neglect and sensory inattention), apraxias (ideomotor, ideational, and constructive), and agnosias present considerable obstacles to successful rehabilitation and to independent living. They present very differently but have been grouped together for this chapter and the level of consciousness, confusion, mood, and motivation also need to be considered and their assessment may include more detail from a clinical psychologist, if appropriate. Table 18.3 gives some investigations which may be of value.

Table 18.3

Cognitive disorders	Appropriate bedside test
Orientation	Hodkinson's test
Memory	Mini-Mental State Examination
Perception	Rivermead behavioural inattention test (star cancellation—(100% sensitivity), line crossing)
Apraxia—ideomotor	Miming simple action, e.g. whistling, combing hair, smiling, waving
Apraxia—ideational	More complex tasks such as miming, lighting candle or cigarette, opening door
Apraxia—constructional	Drawings, building blocks etc. (pick five standard tasks for each problem and simple scores can be derived)
Numeracy	Serial sevens—subtraction from 100
Intellect	Require detailed thorough examination by a clinical psychologist, e.g. IQ, using WAIS-R scale

Some of these tests, such as the Hodkinson's Score, are straightforward. This uses 10 simple questions, one point being scored for each of which can be answered:
- Age of patient
- Address
- Date, month, year
- Name of hospital
- Date of birth
- Name of monarch (or Prime Minister)
- Year of major events
- Ability to count backwards from 20.

A score below 7 suggests a cognitive disorder. The Mini-Mental State examination is a useful screen for memory loss and only takes 5 to 10 minutes to perform. The star cancellation test requires the patient to identify and circle (or cross out) the large stars in the pattern, and visual neglect identifies a pattern where the patient does not appreciate a portion or segment of the figure. Apraxias are essentially an inability to carry out motor tasks, despite having the ability to carry out individual movements. The sequencing of events is at fault and the patient in ideational and constructional apraxias can carry out the individual tasks if cued in to do so. Combining all of them is difficult and often presents considerable problems with independent living. Most resolve within three months of the stroke, but the identification of affected patients is very important. They are often thought of as 'difficult', or 'obstinate' and a sympathetic and informed approach usually provides a much better result. Physiotherapy cannot hope to be successful until these apraxias are managed. All forms of cognitive impairment have a profound effect on the ability of the patient to regain employment, drive a car or live independently.

Special problems

These include incontinence, constipation, and pressure sores, which are all dealt with in other chapters. Pressure sores usually result from immobility and are preventable. The skin over pressure points should therefore be regularly checked in patients with impaired mobility and cognition during their rehabilitation. Side effects of medical treatments can interfere with performance and function, and the use of diuretics and analgesics should be carefully monitored in stroke patients. Spasticity is a major issue in stroke. It is often important to utilize lower limb spasticity early on in the rehabilitation process in order to achieve weight-bearing in weak limbs. Only harmful spasticity requires treatment, and the encouragement of symmetrical weight-bearing will provide the basis of physical treatment of spasticity. Finally, the treatment of depression, as mentioned above, is important.

The process of rehabilitation

There is a vast difference between general rehabilitation and specialist rehabilitation. People with complex disorders (such as communication, cognitive, and sensory deficits, as well as those with comobilities) require the services of a specialized interdisciplinary rehabilitation team where goals are set and agreed, with the full participation of the patient and carers and where achievable targets can be met. Goals for discharge should be made in the context of the overall treatment plan and targets for the final outcome. Obviously, these are subject to change and it is important to stress the continuing nature of the rehabilitation episode. Discharge into the community will depend on a multitude of factors and many units employ specific personnel to ensure that all the patient's needs are met. Full documentation of the rehabilitation treatment is essential and all professionals should not only have access to the clinical notes, but should record their own findings within.

Prediction of outcome

In the context of prognostication, there are predictors of functional outcome. The functional independence measurement, Barthel ADL index and Nottingham ADL index have been validated in stroke and all are ordinal scales, which can be hierarchical, if arranged in an appropriate manner. All are quick and easy to do. The most important outcome, however, is the achievement of the goals set, which can measure the patient's functional progress as well as the accuracy of prognostication and achievability. The success of achieving good quality of life in the community depends on the initial treatment, the integration of specialist-based and community-based rehabilitation services and particularly on non-health issues, over which many doctors have no control. Good and appropriate housing, return to employment, and restoration of occupational and leisure activities are some of the essential measures of success in stroke rehabilitation. However, they are difficult to measure accurately and it is one of the main areas for research.

Conclusions

Stroke is one of the commonest disabling conditions, particularly in the older population. About one-third of

people will die after a stroke within the first month, with
about one-third making a good recovery. This leaves about
one-third of survivors with a significant disability. The
potential range of disabilities is enormous and management
requires the coordinated input of the whole rehabilitation
team. Stroke rehabilitation is now one of the specialist
areas of rehabilitation in which there is convincing
evidence of the efficacy of a coordinated team input and
stroke wards, backed up by community teams, should be a
part of all general hospital services.

Further reading

Warlow, C. P., Dennis, M. S., Van Gijn, K., *et al.* (1996). *Stroke: a
practical guide to management*. Blackwell Scientific, Oxford.

19

....

Head injury

Head injury is probably the most challenging disorder faced by a rehabilitation team. It presents a complicated array of physical, behavioural, emotional, cognitive, and social problems. There is now evidence that outcome following head injury is improved by access to an expert multi-disciplinary team and slowly a number of such teams are emerging in the UK. Head injury rehabilitation needs to be long term. If the individual survives the first few days then, except for a very small proportion of people with major disability, life expectancy is normal. There is now a realization that the rehabilitation team will need to keep in touch with the head injured person and family for many years. Although most benefit follows early intervention there are significant benefits from continuing contact particularly for the prevention of unnecessary physical, psychological, and social complications.

Epidemiology

The annual attendance rate at casualty with head injury is about 1500–2000 per 100 000 population per annum. However, only a quarter or so of these people are admitted to hospital. Even of those who are admitted the majority will have sustained a 'minor' head injury, whereas around

10 per cent will have had a 'moderate' head injury and about 5 per cent a 'severe' head injury. There are significant problems that can follow minor and moderate head injuries (see below) but most of the emphasis of this chapter will be on the more serious consequences that follow from a severe injury to the head and brain. The majority of injuries are from road traffic accidents either as drivers, passengers, or pedestrians. A smaller proportion will be from domestic or industrial accidents or sporting injuries or violence. Prevalence is rather difficult to estimate with accuracy but given the relatively normal life expectancy it is likely that there are 100–150 individuals with a persistent disability as a result of head injury per 100 000 population. Thus, head injury is one of the five most prevalent neurological conditions affecting the central nervous system together with migraine, cerebro-vascular disease, epilepsy, and Parkinson's disease.

Classification and prognosis

The distinction between mild, moderate, and severe head injury can be useful in determining outcome although it is important to emphasize that outcome can be highly variable and unpredictable. There are many individuals who have had a severe head injury with persistent coma for several weeks who regain a totally normal lifestyle just as there are individuals with a mild head injury who have severe persisting problems. Prognosis should never be given in the first few weeks after the accident as significant physical and psychological recovery can take place for at least two years and often longer. A generally accepted classification of head injury relies on the initial Glasgow Coma Score (see Table 19.1), the length of coma, and the length of post-traumatic amnesia. The latter is defined as the period of time from injury until resumption of day-to-day memory. It is difficult to measure in a clinical setting with accuracy and is often a period of time best judged in retrospect. However, the lower the initial Glasgow Coma Score, the greater the length of coma, and the greater the length of post-traumatic amnesia the worse is the long-term prognosis. At the present time there are no more accurate means of determining long-term prognosis. There is a crude correlation between the amount of brain damage (as determined by these measures and also by MRI scanning) and long-term outlook. However, in the short term only crude initial indications or preferably no indication of long-term prognosis should be given. More accurate prognosis can only be determined after the first few months. The majority of physical recovery occurs in the first 12 months (mostly in the first six months) but psychological recovery can occur over a much longer time course of at least two years and sometimes longer. It is important to emphasize these points to relatives in the early stages. Table 19.2 outlines a useful classification of head injury.

Minor head injury

The great majority of people with a minor or moderate head injury make an excellent recovery over a few days. Sometimes there are minor 'post-concussional' symptoms such as headaches, dizziness, insomnia, and fatigue that can persist for several weeks or months but which are of little functional consequence. However, it is increasingly recognized that more subtle but important impairments of cognitive and executive brain function can occur after minor head injuries. There are clearly documented impairments of information-processing speed, attention and concentration, reaction time, and minor memory defects that occur even after the mildest head injury. For many individuals these problems are more of a nuisance than a major problem, but in a significant minority these symptoms can be disabling and can in some people last many months or years. It is important that everyone who has a head injury is given information and advice about possible symptoms which in turn need to be put into the context of their lifestyle. For example, it may be wise for a person operating complicated and potentially dangerous machinery to stay off work if there are problems with concentration and fatigueability until such symptoms pass. Often it is helpful to offer advice to the employers as well as to the

Table 19.1 Glasgow Coma Scale

Item	Response	Score	Details
Eye opening	None	1	Even to pain (supra-orbital pressure)
	To pain	2	Pain from sternum/limb/supra-orbital ridge
	To speech	3	Non-specific response, not necessarily to command
	Spontaneous	4	Eyes open, not necessarily aware
Motor response	None	1	To any pain; limbs remain flaccid
	Extension	2	'Decerebrate'; shoulder adducted and internally rotated, forearm pronated
	Abnormal flexion	3	'Decorticate'; shoulder flexes/adducts
	Withdrawal	4	Arm withdraws from pain, shoulder abducts
	Localizes pain	5	Arm attempts to remove supra-orbital/chest pain
	Obeys commands	6	Follows simple commands
Verbal response	None	1	As stated
	Incomprehensible	2	Moans/groans; no words
	Inappropriate	3	Intelligible, no sustained sentences
	Confused	4	Responds with conversation, but confused
	Oriented	5	Aware of time, place, person

References: Teasdale and Jennett (1974), Teasdale *et al.* (1978, 1979).

Table 19.2 Classification of head injury

Classification	Definition
Mild head injury	Defined as Glasgow Coma Score 13 or 14 Coma < 15 minutes
Moderate head injury	Defined as Glasgow Coma Score 8–12 Coma 15 minutes–6 hours Post-traumatic amnesia < 24 hours
Severe head injury	Defined as Glasgow Coma Score < 7 Coma > 6 hours Post-traumatic amnesia > 24 hours

disabled person and family. It is quite common that individuals with minor head injury return to work too soon and are unable to cope with the job and suffer as a consequence. The logistics of running a mild head injury clinic for everyone who is admitted to a casualty department are probably impossible to cope with in the present National Health Service. However, it should be possible to establish a multidisciplinary clinic at least involving a neurologist and/or rehabilitation physician and clinical neuropsychologist for all those who have persisting symptoms after say three months. Such a clinic could deal with the medical and psychosocial issues and help the individual establish appropriate coping strategies as well as providing advice, information, and liaison with community services. Such clinics are extremely rare world-wide.

Organization of head injury services

It is well known that secondary brain damage can occur after primary head injury, particularly as a result of oedema and anoxia. Fast emergency care and appropriate treatment of other injuries is vital and the best outcome is probably obtained by immediate transfer to a trauma centre for stabilization. Such centres should ideally be in close association with a neurosurgical unit specializing in head injury with access to MRI scanning facilities and cerebral pressure monitoring. It is outside the scope of this book to deal with the acute neurosurgical management of head injury. However, the rehabilitation team should be associated with the acute neurosurgical team as soon as possible. There are a number of complications that can arise in the first few hours and days after injury which if properly dealt with can save major rehabilitation problems later. Two examples would be active intervention for spasticity in order to prevent contractures and an assessment of swallowing with appropriate initiation of intravenous or gastrostomy feeding.

As soon as the individual is surgically stable, transfer to a rehabilitation centre should be organized. If the rehabilitation unit is geared to cope then transfer even at the stage of coma or in the phase of post-traumatic amnesia is still important in order that passive rehabilitation can take place, particularly to prevent unnecessary physical complications. For example, on a neurosurgical unit it is often necessary for major behavioural problems to be treated with sedation for fear of disturbance or harm to other vulnerable people. This is usually unhelpful in the long term and can be better managed in an appropriately designed and staffed head injury rehabilitation unit. There is now no doubt that there are better functional outcomes, often shorter length of stay, better provision of information and support to the carers and family, and clear psychological benefit from admission to a dedicated head injury rehabilitation unit.

Common problems after severe head injury

Physical disability

Fortunately severe physical disability following head injury is quite uncommon. However, avoidance of complications, particularly in the early stages during recovery, is vital in order to maximize the chance of a good recovery. Early therapy should emphasize the importance of prevention of contractures and the management of spasticity. Proper attention to positioning and seating is vital.

Standing in a standing frame or tilt table is useful, and there is some evidence that this can reduce the risk of osteoporosis and later risk of fracture. Range of motion exercises are important as well as the use of splints and casts, sometimes in combination with peripheral nerve or motor blocks or botulinum injections (see Chapter 6). Later there is more emphasis on retraining of movement control and coordination. Although early intervention is vital it is also important to emphasize the value of later and ongoing intervention with the use of a tailored exercise programme.

Obviously traumatic brain injury can affect any part of the central nervous system. Thus there is a plethora of potential physical complications. Commonly such problems will include communication difficulties, swallowing problems, continence problems, and obviously difficulties with activities of daily living in association with arm dysfunction. The treatment and rehabilitation potential of such problems are outlined in the appropriate chapters in this book.

Prolonged coma and vegetative state

A few individuals regrettably remain in prolonged coma (defined as coma of more than two weeks' duration) or in a persistent vegetative state. Prognosis in such individuals is obviously poor but nevertheless longer-term improvements are possible. In one study about half of those patients who were still unaware at one month subsequently regained awareness and of those about three-quarters eventually returned home, albeit with severe residual disabilities. Only around 10 per cent of those recovering consciousness returned to gainful employment. Some units use sensory stimulation to try to reduce the length of coma, but there is, so far, no definite evidence that such techniques have benefit. Recently there have been case reports of some recovery after unconsciousness lasting several years. These individuals have recovered to a very dependent state but nevertheless these cases demonstrate the moral dilemma of withdrawing active support from those in prolonged coma. It is now recommended that such decisions should never be taken before one year and many authorities would now say that such decisions should be delayed for at least two years. There are significant nursing and therapy challenges in preventing complications in those with prolonged coma and transfer to a specialist unit is desirable.

Cognitive impairments

There are a variety of important cognitive impairments that can follow a head injury. These are covered in more detail in Chapter 15. The commonest problems are associated with attention, concentration, memory, perception, information-processing speed, and problem solving. The first task is a proper assessment of the extent of the impairment and consequent disability by a clinical neuropsychologist. Natural recovery can take place over a prolonged period and real progress is often seen up to two years post-injury. It is controversial whether neuropsychological interventions can actually promote such recovery, but there is no doubt that coping strategies can be designed which effectively reduce disability. It is possible that some neuropsychological interventions can have a direct effect on the impairment itself, although controlled experimentation in this field is fraught with problems. Single case studies are, however, now beginning to show the efficacy of some interventions. It is important that a hospital-based programme is able to generalize into normal life and obviously such intervention should be designed to have an impact on disability and quality of life rather than simply have an impact on an artificial neuropsychological measurement instrument.

Behavioural problems

Behavioural problems are extremely common in the early recovery phase following head injury, particularly where the individual is still in post-traumatic amnesia. A small number of people will develop significant long-term behavioural problems.

Sedative or psychotropic medication should be avoided. Such medication will simply add to confusion when the drug effects begin to wear off necessitating further drug administration and so on. In the longer term cognitive and behavioural management techniques are effective in ameliorating difficult behaviour. This has been demonstrated even several years after injury. However, such techniques are difficult to put into practice except in specialist units as all staff and relatives will need to cooperate in a strict behavioural regime. Behavioural management for severe ongoing problems can take several months to have any longer-term, generalizable effect. Further details of behavioural management techniques are outlined in Chapter 13.

Personality and emotional problems

These changes are often most frequently reported by relatives. It is common to hear the comment 'he is not the man I married' or 'it is like living with a different person'. 'Personality change' is an unhelpful term. It is better to document the details of any perceived change in order to provide information and hopefully design some form of coping strategy. Changes can be many and include childish behaviour, fatuousness, egocentricity, irritability, aggressiveness, lack of initiation and reduced drive, lethargy, lack of social skills, and increased or decreased sexual interest. These changes can obviously lead to major problems within the marriage, family, and wider social circles, particularly in employment. Clinical depression or anxiety are quite common at some point during the recovery phase. Occasionally more profound psychiatric problems can be seen such as psychosis, mania, or obsessive compulsive disorder. Most of these psychiatric disorders are amenable to standard therapy. A neuropsychiatrist is a useful associated team member in addition to the continuing input from the neuropsychologist. More subtle personality changes are certainly difficult to ameliorate. Counselling or formal psychotherapy has been advocated, although there is little evidence to confirm effectiveness. Often it is regrettably a matter of information to the family members and employers in order to help them cope better with a very difficult home and work situation. Support to the carers in terms of information, counselling, advice, and practical help at home, including respite breaks, are as important as direct assistance to the head injured individual.

Later rehabilitation

In the longer term retraining of independent living skills and social skills become more important. There may be a need for ongoing behavioural management for inappropriate social behaviour. There is emerging evidence of the efficacy of specific retraining for memory and social skills as well as independent living skills such as cooking, shopping, and community mobility. There now a number of so-called transitional living units or tertiary rehabilitation units that specialize in this area, although it is fair to say that there is so far only limited evidence of the generalizability of such retraining programmes. In the later stages the involvement of a wide range of health, social service, and employment professionals is often required. Access and coordination of all these different professionals can be a major problem for the disabled person and their family. In legal settlements it is now common for a case manager to be appointed who can assist with such coordination and often act as an advocate for the family.

Recently, at least in the UK, there has been increased investment in head injury rehabilitation. The emergence of post-acute head injury rehabilitation units should produce early functional benefit but longer-term support by this team or by a parallel community team is equally important to ensure both disability and handicap are kept to a minimum for this important group of disabled people.

Conclusions

Head injury is common. The majority of people will sustain only a minor head injury but nevertheless even after minor injuries there is still a significant range of problems in the short term and for some in the long term. Those with more severe injuries have a whole plethora of physical, cognitive, behavioural, and emotional problems and present one of the most significant challenges to a rehabilitation team.

There is now emerging evidence that a coordinated, multidisciplinary, and specialist rehabilitation team can produce sustainable functional benefit in the acute phase and into the longer term. In many ways the problems of head injury epitomize the whole range of difficulties encountered by disabled people. A good head injury service should provide a model for a good general disability service.

Further reading

Ashley, M. J. and Krych, D. K. (1995). *Traumatic brain injury rehabilitation*. CRC Press, Boca Raton, FL.

Chamberlain, M. A., Neumann, V., and Tennant, A. (1995). *Traumatic brain injury rehabilitation*. Chapman and Hall, London.

Finlayson, M. A. J. and Garner, S. H. (1994). *Brain injury rehabilitation: clinical considerations*. Williams and Wilkins, Baltimore.

Hubert, J. (1995). *Life after head injury*. Avebury, Aldershot.

Levin, H. S., Eisenberg, H. M., and Benton, A. L. (1989). *Mild head injury*. Oxford University Press, Oxford.

McMillan, T. M. and Greenwood, R. J. (1993). Head injury. In: Greenwood, R., Barnes, M. P., McMillan, T. M., and Ward, C. D. (ed.) *Neurological rehabilitation*, pp.437–50. Churchill Livingstone, London.

Ponsford, J. (1996). *Traumatic brain injury: rehabilitation for everyday adaptive living*. Psychology Press, Hove.

Powell, T. (1995). *Head injury: a practical guide*. Headway National Head Injuries Association /Winslow Press, Nottingham and Bicester.

Teasdale, G. and Jennett, B. (1974). Assessment of coma and impaired consciousness. A practical scale. *Lancet*, **2**, 81–3.

Teasdale, G., Knill-Jones, R., and Van der Sande, J. (1978). Observer variability in assessing impaired consciousness and coma. *Journal of Neurology, Neurosurgery and Psychiatry*, **41**, 603–10.

Teasdale, G., Murray, G., Parker, L., and Jennett, B. (1979). Adding up the Glasgow Coma Scale. *Acta Neurochirurgica*, Suppl 28, 13–16.

20

....

Spinal injury

There have been huge advances in the rehabilitation of people with spinal injuries over the last few decades. Those with spinal injuries during World War I had an 80 per cent mortality rate within three years. The major cause of death was urinary tract infection or complications from pressure sores and limb contractures. Now the overall life expectancy is virtually normal, except for the few people with very high cervical cord injuries and ventilator dependence. Advances in both acute management and rehabilitation techniques have largely been responsible for this dramatic improvement.

Incidence and causation

In the UK there are about 15–20 cases of traumatic spinal cord injury per million population per annum. The commonest causes in this country are road traffic accidents, which account for approximately half of all cases, followed by domestic and industrial falls and sporting injuries. Males are three times more likely to be injured than females and the most frequently injured age group are those between 20 and 40 years. Obviously causation varies significantly world-wide. In many parts of the tropics the commonest cause are falls from trees or down wells whilst in the United States a significant cause is gun-shot injury. In recent conflicts in ex-Yugoslavia the commonest cause has been sniper injury. The distribution of injury is approximately equal between the cervical spine, more commonly at lower cervical levels, and the thoraco-lumbar spine. However, it should be remembered that in about 8 per cent of people the spine is injured at more than one level.

Pathophysiology

The majority of damage occurs at the time of impact, often with direct tissue and neural trauma. However, there are a number of secondary vascular, biochemical, and electrolyte changes producing further haemorrhage, infarction, oedema, neuronal injury, or death. Some of these factors are potentially reversible either naturally or with intervention. Thus, although neural recovery can generally be predicted by the initial extent of injury there is the uncertainty of the potentially reversible element and definitive prognosis, which should never be given in the early stages. It is likely that in the next few years there will be some progress made towards direct promotion of neural recovery by means of neural transplantation or the use or manipulation of various neuro-modulatory and nerve growth factors. However, at this time there is no intervention that is known to promote natural recovery, with the possible exception of adminis-tration of high-dose methyl prednisolone given within eight hours of injury.

Acute management

The basic objective of either surgical or medical manage-ment of spinal injury is to reduce a displaced fracture, stabilize the unstable injury, and restore or at least preserve neurological function. It is outside the scope of this textbook to discuss the acute and initial surgical manage-ment of spinal cord injuries. However, successful rehabilitation must begin at the scene of the accident to be sure there are as few complications as possible. The airway, breathing, and circulation should be monitored and the individual immobilized prior to transfer. Transfer to the nearest trauma centre is probably associated with a better outcome, particularly if there are other life-threatening injuries. However, either directly or as soon as possible after initial trauma management the individual should be transferred to a centre with expertise in spinal cord injury. There is no doubt that eventual functional recovery is maximized by rehabilitation being carried out in such centres.

There is considerable debate in spinal injury circles regarding the relative merits of conservative management as opposed to surgical management of the fracture. The basis for conservative treatment is fracture reduction and bed rest until the injury is stable after which the individual can be mobilized with or without external fixation. Cervical injuries can be reduced by cervical traction using skull callipers. However, whilst most fractures will unite and become stable the average period of time to do so is around 10 weeks. This period of bed rest can have many adverse psychological and physical consequences. Cervical traction itself is not without some risk from, for example, over distraction and infection of the pin sites. Surgical stabilization will allow earlier mobilization and facilitate nursing care and allow earlier access to a full rehabilitation programme. The degree of neurological recovery is similar whether surgical or conservative management is undertaken. The overall problems of prolonged immobilization on the one hand and surgical risk on the other about balance each other out in terms of undesirable complications.

Assessment of potential

The most important factor is the neurological level of injury and the completeness or incompleteness of function below that level. Obviously incomplete lesions have a better prognosis for functional recovery than complete lesions.

The following general guide-lines will indicate possible functional outcomes of various spinal levels.

C1–4 level

The main concern with spinal injuries at this level is the likelihood of phrenic nerve involvement and diaphragm paralysis, with additional respiratory problems from weak neck and intercostal muscles. The individual is likely to be ventilator dependent. However, some people can be managed with implanted phrenic nerve pace makers. Others will be permanently ventilator dependent and eventually require home ventilation. The individuals will be quadriplegic and thus will have an important need for environmental control equipment and specialist wheel-chairs. Environmental control equipment can be operated by a suck/puff device and very recently voice activated equipment has also become available. Control of equipment by eye movement is also now technically feasible. Robotic equipment is also now beginning to enter the market place. Powered wheelchairs are available that can be operated by breath control, chin control, head control, or voice activation depending on the exact ability that remains. However, it is very likely that the individual will require some assistance from a third party for virtually all activities of daily living.

C5 level

Individuals with a C5 level injury will have a functional deltoid and/or biceps muscle. This can, with appropriate splinting, allow some useful arm functions. A forearm orthosis can make arm placement easier for such activities as feeding and typing and an orthosis with slots for utensils and pens can provide wrist stability and can also aid with feeding, writing, and typing. Most people with C5 lesions can feed themselves, perform simple oral and facial hygiene and offer some assistance with upper-half dressing. However, it is likely that a powered wheelchair will still be needed although some people can just manage a manual wheelchair with a hand rim, particularly for propelling indoors and on smooth surfaces.

C6 level

At C6 level active wrist extension becomes possible as well as some degree of hand function although orthoses are usually still required often with utensil slots and pen holders. People at this level can usually feed themselves when food is cut up, perform oral and facial hygiene and upper-half dressing independently. Usually some assistance is required for lower-half dressing. There is often sufficient independence to allow for self-catheterization and performance of some degree of anal cleansing, perhaps with the assistive devices. Manual wheelchair propelling is generally possible, as is driving with appropriate adaptations.

C7/8 level

At this point a functional triceps is added which can greatly improve transfer, mobility, and upper arm skills. At this level most activities of daily living are independent and active elbow extension facilitates wheelchair skills. At C8 flexor digitorum profundus usually becomes functional and although the hand is not normal there is nearly always useful and practical function such that the individual is effectively only paraplegic from this level downwards.

Thoracic levels

The T1 level is the first level with normal hand function, and as the level descends caudally intercostal abdominal muscles recover. This allows for improved respiratory function and trunk balance. People at all thoracic levels should be independent, albeit in a wheelchair, and should be able to manage their bowel and bladder functions. There are a number of orthotic devices that allow for paraplegic ambulation, including standard metal upright knee ankle foot orthoses (KAFO), advanced types of reciprocating gait orthoses (RGO), and hip guidance orthoses (HGO). These devices, sometimes combined with functional neuromuscular stimulation, have demonstrated that ambulation is possible at these spinal levels but it is uncommon for individuals to be community ambulators. However, there are significant rejection rates with such orthoses, probably because of the high energy expenditure required.

Lumbar levels

At the lumbar levels individuals are usually entirely independent and can ambulate without a wheelchair. Hip flexion is present at the L2 level, knee extension at L3, and ankle dorsi flexion at L4. L5 adds extensor hallucis longus and the S1 level adds the gastrocnemius and soleus muscles.

Rehabilitation management

Rehabilitation management should start on day one and even in the immobilization or post-operative phase proper attention must be given to skin care, respiratory care, urinary and bowel care, management of spasticity, and prevention of contractures as well as the necessary levels of information, counselling, and psychological support. More active rehabilitation will obviously start once the individual is able to mobilize and is surgically stable.

Mobility and activities of daily living

We have already seen the complex range of mobility equipment that is necessary according to spinal level. A chin- or head-controlled electric wheelchair being needed for the high cervical quadriplegic and manual wheelchairs being possible from C6 downwards. Functional gait becomes a possibility at a lower thoracic level with modern orthoses and independent ambulation increasingly possible at the lumbar levels. There are now a bewildering variety of wheelchairs available and the new UK government wheelchair voucher scheme will add to the choice of possible chairs. Advice from a rehabilitation physician, physiotherapist, occupational therapist, and orthotist is essential for all those with spinal cord injuries. A rehabilitation engineer can be a particularly valuable member of the team, especially for those people with higher cervical levels whose quality of life and independence can be promoted by a variety of custom-made devices. Modern environmental control equipment is particularly important for promoting independence and this can now be used by those with the highest cervical levels.

Urinary tract

Access to urological advice and urodynamics is essential in any spinal injury rehabilitation programme. If not treated properly urinary infection and eventual renal damage can still lead to morbidity and early death. In the first few days after spinal injury there is usually a period described as spinal shock with a flaccid bladder, managed by an indwelling catheter. Usually this phase is then superseded by a period of detrusor over-activity with resulting urgency and urge incontinence often complicated by detrusor sphincter dysynergia (see Chapter 7). Residual urine should be avoided as this will tend to lead to persistent urinary infection. Normally self-intermittent catheterization is preferable or failing that long-term supra-pubic drainage is often required. Uninhibited detrusor activity can be controlled to some extent by anti-cholinergic medication or occasionally by surgical intervention or more recently by injection of botulinum toxin. A urodynamic assessment including videocystourography is necessary to make a proper assessment of bladder function. A variety of other surgical procedures including anterior sacral root stimulation are now possible and are discussed in more detail in Chapter 7. Long-term monitoring by the rehabilitation team, and preferably by the urological service, remains essential for life.

Autonomic function

Autonomic dysreflexia is a potentially fatal complication of spinal injury which is characterized by an exaggerated autonomic response to a stimulus or stimuli that are innocuous to the able bodied person. People with injuries above T6 are at most risk of such problems. The incidence ranges widely from around 50 to 80 per cent of those at risk and most cases occur between two months and 12 months post-injury, but can occur later. The dysreflexia results from noxious stimuli below the level of the lesion. Distension of the pelvic organs such as the bladder, colon, or rectum, induce sympathetic activity resulting in vasoconstriction and hypertension. There is an exaggerated response to noradrenaline released as a result of the lack of supra-spinal vasomotor reflexes. Other stimuli include catheterization, urinary infections, sexual intercourse, pressure ulcers, and even tight clothing, shoes, or leg bags. Surgical procedures are another common cause of the syndrome. Symptoms include headache, sweating, vasodilatation, nasal obstruction, paraesthesia, and anxiety. There is often significant hypertension. Awareness of the problem and relief of the primary cause are the main treatments. Otherwise attention is directed to a reduction in blood pressure. Sublingual nifedepine can be used or in more severe cases intravenous hydralazine. Chlorpromazine, nitroprusside, and diazoxide are also possibilities. In recent cases alpha-blockers or ganglionic blockers such as phenoxybenzamine or guanethidine have been used.

Pain and dysaesthesia

Peripheral pain is common in the early weeks after injury. Unfortunately burning pain can continue for some months after injury. It is usually well treated by the use of carbamazepine or by the tricyclic anti-depressants. Pain from other sources, such as osteoarthritis, can always occur but it must be remembered that people with spinal cord injury sometimes do not appreciate pain or it is manifested in different ways, such as autonomic dysreflexia or worsening of spasticity. For example, a fall from a chair causing a fractured femur can yield no pain at all and only be manifest by swelling of the leg or worsening of spasticity.

Nutrition and bowels

In the early catabolic stages of recovery a high-protein and high-calorie diet is required. However, eventually the individual will need a good-quality high-fibre diet to maintain health and weight. Despite problems with neural control of bowel function most individuals do achieve reflex bowel emptying on a regular basis either using suppositories or digital anal stimulation. Occasionally regular enemas are required.

Sexual function and fertility

Spinal injury can damage the normal control of the sexual organs and can obviously cause problems for full enjoyment of sexual activity. In addition positioning may be a problem and there is a risk of autonomic dysreflexia. In the male if there is an intact sacral neural loop reflex erections can occur which are sometimes sufficient to achieve intercourse. However, ejaculation is rarer. Despite these problems sexual satisfaction should be entirely possible and is often achieved by non-genital sexual activity. Advice from a sexual therapist or appropriately trained counsellor or psychologist is invaluable. There are various methods to achieve erection in the male (see Chapter 8). Fertility is usually maintained in both the male and female although the quality of semen in the male is sometimes not adequate for fertilization. Emission of semen can be obtained by use of a vibrator either used at the root of the penis or by transrectal electrostimulation. *In vitro* fertilization and other fertility techniques can be used with success. The process of pregnancy and delivery in the female should be straightforward although there is always the risk of autonomic dysreflexia. Management should normally be in a obstetric unit familiar with the problems of spinal cord injured people.

Other medical problems

Deep venous thrombosis
Deep venous thrombosis (DVT) is a major complication after spinal injury and there is a small risk of death from

pulmonary embolism. Conservative management of the injury and prolonged immobilization is an added risk. Heparin is the best prophylactic. External pneumatic calf compression can also be used.

Heterotopic ossification

This is a term that is used when bone develops in an abnormal anatomical position in soft tissues. The prevalence in spinal cord injury is reported to be between 5 and 50 per cent. It most commonly occurs around the hips and the knees although other joints can be involved. The problem causes a decreased range of movement in the joint as well as localized swelling, warmth, and joint effusion. It usually occurs in the first few months after injury and is unusual to begin later than one year post-injury. Treatment is very difficult. Etidromate disodium (didronel) is the most useful treatment. It probably does not prevent ossification but the amount of bone deposited would seem to be less. In severe cases surgical intervention can be required but surgery is generally unsatisfactory. Some centres now use etidromate disodium prophylactically for about a year.

Spasticity and contractures

Spasticity is extremely common after spinal injury and if not properly treated can progress to contracture. Some spasticity can be functionally useful and can, for example, be used as an aid to standing in individuals with low-level lesions or as an aid to dressing when putting on trousers. Treatment focuses on proper seating and positioning supplemented by various anti-spastic physiotherapy techniques and the judicial use of orthoses. Oral anti-spastic medication can be helpful although side effects tend to limit dosage. Focal treatment with phenol nerve blocks or intramuscular botulinum toxin are very helpful methods. Rarely intrathecal baclofen or other surgical techniques such as rhizotomies can be used in more advanced cases. If spasticity is untreated and contractures form then occasionally surgery is the only way to get a useful relief of symptoms in order to ease positioning and nursing care. Further details on the management of spasticity are discussed in Chapter 6.

Respiratory problems

Unfortunately pneumonia is still a leading cause of morbidity and death after spinal injury. Although inter-costal muscles and abdominal muscles contribute to respiration the major muscle used in respiration is the diaphragm. Thus, the main risk in spinal cord injury is the involvement of the phrenic nerve in high cervical lesions. Phrenic nerve stimulation is a relatively new technique and can be used with success in some indi-viduals. Other methods include the use of an abdominal binder in order to elevate the diaphragm to a higher, more functional resting position. Proper wheelchair positioning in order to prevent chest deformity, use of glosopharyngeal breathing (frog breathing) to improve vital capacity and assist with cough can be useful. Other physiotherapy techniques such as simple deep-breathing exercises and exercises to increase thoracic expansion, strength, and intercostal muscles are also used. In high cervical lesions respiratory ventilator support will be necessary and it is now quite possible for individuals to have portable ventilators for use at home or even attached to a wheel-chair.

Pressure sores

Pressure sores are a risk in immobile people but never-theless should be preventable. Proper seating and cushioning are the most important preventative factors. Individuals will often require special wheelchair cushion-ing such as a Jay cushion or RoHo cushion. Individuals are usually taught to 'lift' if possible using their arms on the wheelchair at frequent intervals in order to relieve pressure. Pressure relieving mattresses may be required at night. The individual and their main carer should be taught to monitor the skin carefully and immediately take pressure off an area that shows persistent redness, a sign of imminent breakdown. Once present pressure sores are very difficult to treat adequately and often require a long period of hospitalization, often combined with plastic surgery. Unfortunately pressure sores and subse-quent sepsis are still a cause of death in spinal cord injury.

Organization of services

The complex array of potential problems following spinal injury require the input of a trained and experienced multidisciplinary team. There is clear evidence that better functional outcomes in spinal injury are obtained if the individual is transferred as soon as possible to an appropriate spinal centre. In the UK spinal centres are, for historical reasons, usually separate from other rehabilitation units. Few units are able to have the totally comprehensive range of expertise and there is a recent trend to combine spinal units with broader-based regional rehabilitation centres. Such centres are likely to contain a full complement of staff, including psychology and counselling, and a broader range of facilities such as a driving assessment centre. Other services will need to be accessed by the centre including employment rehabilitation and social work and preferably the local branch of the Spinal Injuries Association for peer support and advice.

Conclusions

Although traumatic spinal cord injury is quite rare it is vital that such people have access to a specialist rehabilitation team. There are quite specific problems associated with spinal cord injury. This particularly includes a range of problems associated with the urinary tract, autonomic dysfunction, sexual dysfunction, and an important need for psychological support for people who have a serious physical disability but with preserved cognition and intellect.

Further reading

ABC of spinal cord injury (1996). British Medical Journal Publications, London.

Aisen, M. L. (1994). Spinal cord injury. In: Good, D. C. and Couch, J. R. (ed.) *Neurological rehabilitation*, pp.561–84. Marcel Dekker, New York,

Berkowitz, M., Harvey, C., Greene, C. G., and Wilson, S. E. (1992). *The economic consequences of traumatic spinal cord injury.* Demos, New York.

Dobkin, B. H. (1996). *Neurological rehabilitation*, pp.218–56. F. A. Davis, Philadelphia.

Yarkony, G. M. (ed.) (1994). *Spinal cord injury—medical management of rehabilitation.* Rehabilitation Institute of Chicago Procedure Manuals, Aspen, MD.

21

....

Parkinson's disease and movement disorders

Parkinson's disease

In the last 25 years there have been huge improvements in the drug therapy of Parkinson's disease such that, at least in the early stages, disability and handicap can be kept to an absolute minimum. However, in the later stages there is less satisfactory response to dopaminergic therapy and major problems of disability and handicap can arise presenting significant challenges to the rehabilitation team.

Causes of Parkinsonism

It is important to emphasize that there are a large number of other causes of Parkinsonism (see Table 21.1). Some of these may be treatable by appropriate intervention for the primary disease (e.g. Wilson's disease) or removal of the offending agent such as for drug-induced Parkinsonism. However, many of the other forms of Parkinsonism, particularly the Parkinson's plus syndromes and multiple system atrophies, remain resistant to drug therapy.

An accurate diagnosis is essential in order to give a prognosis and to plan an appropriate treatment and rehabilitation strategy.

Table 21.1 Causes of Parkinsonism

Class of disorder	Manifestation
Degenerative diseases	Parkinson's disease
	Progressive supra nuclear palsy
	Multiple system atrophies
	Olivopontocerebellar atrophy
Infections	Post encephalitic Parkinsonism
Drug or toxin induced	Neuroleptics
	Carbon monoxide poisoning
	Manganese poisoning
	MPTP induced Parkinsonism
Vascular conditions	Vascular conditions
	Hypertensive encephalopathy
Trauma	Head injury
	Punch drunk syndrome
Cerebral tumour	
Other neurological conditions that may have Parkinsonian features	Alzheimer's disease
	Intermittently raised pressure hydrocephalus
	Various forms of Huntington's disease
	Wilson's disease

Epidemiology

Parkinson's disease is one of the commoner neurological disabling conditions. The prevalence is approximately 150–200 per 100 00 population in the UK with an incidence of about 18–20 per 100 000 population per annum. The male/female ratio is 3:2. The disorder becomes more common as age progresses and approximately one in 10 people over the age of 80 have Parkinsonism. However, the mean age of onset is 55 years and so the disorder is not exclusively a problem of the elderly and will often occur in individuals who are still economically active.

Principal features

The four leading features of Parkinson's disease are brady-kinesia, rigidity, tremor, and impairment of postural reflexes.

Bradykinesia

Bradykinesia is a term that describes slowness of voluntary movement including delay in initiation and execution of the movement. Early manifestations are common in the hands resulting in impairment of fine-skilled tasks, such as writing. It may be increasingly difficult to button clothing or use cutlery. At the same time associated movements such as arm swing and facial expression are often reduced. The latter can given rise to diagnostic confusion with depression.

Rigidity

Rigidity is the term that describes resistant to passive muscle stretch classically described as either 'lead pipe' or 'plastic'. Rigidity is present in the trunk muscles as well as the limb muscles and is the feature that gives rise to the characteristic stooped posture. A combination of brady-kinesia and rigidity are the two features that cause the most disablement.

Tremor

Tremor in Parkinson's disease is usually a slow rest tremor. However, occasionally other forms of tremor are seen, such as action or postural tremor. The tremor is usually an embarrassment rather than a functional problem, at least in the early stages.

Impaired postural reflexes

In many of the Parkinsonian syndromes it is often difficult to maintain balance due to impairment of postural reflexes. This causes stumbling, particularly in busy streets or when trying to hurry or change direction.

Medical management

The mainstay of treatment in Parkinson's disease is dopa replacement therapy. The commonest mode of treatment is for direct levodopa replacement combined with carbidopa—a peripheral decarboxylase inhibitor—that reduces peripheral side effects. There are now various combinations of carbidopa/levodopa as well as controlled release and other preparations. It is often a matter of trial and error to find the right balance of tablet combinations. In general the best mode of administration is usually to give a smaller dose at frequent intervals throughout the day. The minimum dose compatible with the desired reduction in symptom levels is a good guide-line. This may mean that the treatment has to be more aggressive in the younger person who is still at work and needs a reasonable degree of control and coordination whereas treatment can be less aggressive in the older person who simply needs to get around the house adequately. There has been a long debate in neurological circles about the best time to start treatment. Some authorities would start as soon as the diagnosis is made while others would wait as late as possible so that complications of treatment are delayed as long as possible. A useful guide-line is to initiate treatment as and when the symptoms become troublesome and interfere with the level of activity required by that individual. This may mean early intervention for the young active person and much later intervention for the minimally disabled elderly person.

A variety of other methods of treatment are now available. Some would start first with dopamine agonist agents, such as bromocriptine, pergolide, lysuride, cabergoline, or ropinerole. Others would use these agents as second-line drugs in combination with levodopa. Selegiline (a dopamine B-oxidase inhibitor) is thought to slow progression of the disease and was widely used until a few years ago when studies indicated doubts about long-term efficacy and safety. Anti-cholinergic agents have a variety of undesirable side effects, particularly confusion, dry mouth, blurred vision, constipation, and impaired erection, but nevertheless can be useful treatments, particularly for troublesome tremor.

Although dopamine replacement therapy is extremely effective in the short term eventually treatment problems arise. These usually occur after 5–10 years. The individual can begin to swing from a rigid phase ('off') to a phase of marked dyskinetic movements ('on'). This on/off swinging can take a variety of patterns and the dosage and timing of the treatment become increasingly problematic. A recent advance is the use of self-injected apomorphine which is a direct-acting D_1 dopamine agonist but with rapid onset of action. A single injection can be used to rescue people from a bad 'off' period.

The other forms of Parkinsonism can be treated by a similar regime of dopamine replacement but response to treatment, particularly in the Parkinson plus syndromes, is usually very poor. Thus, prognosis in terms of survival and disability in these syndromes is worse than in Parkinson's disease.

Disabling features of Parkinson's disease

Gait

The most immediate problem in Parkinson's disease is the shuffling and insecure gait which can cause frequent falls. Bradykinesia and rigidity are largely responsible combined with impaired postural reflexes and often compounded by troublesome and severe dyskinetic movements as a result of treatment. Advice from a physiotherapist can be helpful, even in the early stages. Various trick strategies can be taught to overcome the problem of initiation of movement and freezing. For example, rising from a chair can be difficult and the individual can be taught to rock backwards and forwards until there is sufficient momentum to rise up. Freezing can sometimes be helped by getting the patient to pretend that they have to step up over a small obstruction. Rigid muscles can be uncomfortable and stretching exercises are often found to be helpful. It is unlikely that physiotherapy can improve bradykinesia and rigidity *per se* but a number of studies have now confirmed the psychological and social value of physiotherapy guided exercises, particularly in a group setting. Early referral to physiotherapy with repeated short pulses of intensive treatment is preferable to late referral.

Activities of daily living

The same problems with bradykinesia, rigidity, and tremor will often cause problems with fine hand and arm movements. Once again it is unlikely that intervention, for example by a physiotherapist or occupational therapist, can actually improve the underlying problem but functional benefit can follow from prescription of suitable aids. Large-handled cutlery, plate guards, use of Velcro instead of buttons, and aids to writing are but a few examples of the value of a proper occupational therapy assessment.

Speech and swallowing

Characteristic changes of speech are often described as dysarthrophonia—a combination of problems with both articulation and phonation. It is characterized by a monotonous pitch and quietness of articulation with the words often coming in short rushes at variable rates due to impaired breath control. Stuttering can also be a problem. Dysphagia is quite common. Overall, early referral to a speech and language therapist is helpful. A recent study demonstrated that appropriate speech exercises produced significant improvements in intonation, stress, and rhythm in the early stages. However, in more advanced cases when communication is almost impossible the speech therapist is also the best person to advise on various forms of augmentative communication (see Chapter 10). The speech therapist, often in combination with a dietician and radiologist, is best placed to organize a proper swallowing assessment (see Chapter 9). Such assessment can be followed by advice on posture, relaxation, food consistency and texture, and nutritional content, all of which can ease the distressing problem of dysphagia and increasing malnutrition.

Autonomic problems

Postural hypotension can be found in Parkinson's disease but is commoner in the associated syndromes, particularly Shy–Drager syndrome. Treatment is remarkably difficult. Advice on avoiding rapid changes of posture, large meals, excessive alcohol, warm temperatures, and excessive straining might be adequate in mild cases. Compressive garments, such as elastic stockings and abdominal binders, can be worn in more extreme cases but are often impractical and of little benefit. Fludrocortisone treatment is probably the best therapy but only has limited success.

Bladder difficulties are remarkably common occurring in approximately 50 per cent of people with Parkinson's disease and often take the form of frequency, urgency, or urge incontinence although sometimes hesitancy and retention are problems. Appropriate treatment is outlined in Chapter 7. Constipation is also common but can usually be overcome by an appropriate diet and a regular pattern of defecation.

Pain

Pain is quite a common problem in Parkinson's disease and unfortunately is under recognized and poorly treated. Pain is often due to the cramp-like pains associated with muscle rigidity and as such is best treated by appropriate anti-Parkinsonian medication. However, in an ageing population additional pain can result from osteoarthritis and will thus need a different approach.

Sleep disorders

Sleep disorders are remarkably common in Parkinson's disease. The commonest problem is so-called 'sleep fragmentation' characterized by recurrent waking, often in turn due to joint pains, intermittent rigidity or tremor, or the inability to turn over at night because of bradykinesia. Daytime fatigue is consequently common. Trial and error with late-night medication can produce some benefit.

Devices to help turn over in bed, such as a strap on the bed head to hold on to or even the very simple device of wearing cotton beds socks to give some further purchase on the sheets, can occasionally produce gratifying results. If at all possible night sedation should be avoided as this often worsens the daytime somnolence and causes additional and unnecessary side effects in a person already on an often complicated therapeutic regime.

Sexual function

The literature on sexuality in Parkinson's disease is remarkably sparse. It is likely that the disorder itself can cause problems as a result of autonomic dysfunction. Drug intervention, particularly anticholinergics, can cause additional problems. Physical impairments can cause mechanical difficulties during sex. The situation can often be helped by advice on posture, alternative means of sexual stimulation, and perseverance with appropriate drug timing. Counselling can be helpful, particularly if there are problems with self image and relationships.

Cognitive and emotional state

Depression is common in Parkinson's disease and is reported in about half of all cases. Depression, as in any chronic neurological disorder, should be treated aggressively and there is no evidence of any different response to intervention when compared with idiopathic depression (see Chapter 14). There is now extensive literature on the incidence of dementia and cognitive impairment in Parkinson's disease. The eventual incidence of dementia has been widely estimated to be between 10 and 80%. Dementia is often characterized by a change in behaviour towards dependency, indecision, and passivity. Even in the absence of overt dementia more subtle cognitive defects are often found, including memory problems, perseveration, and difficulties with information-processing speed. An assessment by a neuropsychologist can be helpful. Cognitive defects are often compounded by the associated problems of the ageing brain, particularly increasing forgetfulness.

Issues in service delivery

It is clear that a team approach is essential in the overall management of Parkinson's disease and Parkinsonism. A neurologist or geriatrician is often involved in the medical management and a case can be made for a specific Parkinson's clinic which in turn can be supported by appropriate therapists. A recent model is the development of the Parkinson's disease nurse practitioner who, with special training, can advise individuals on drug management as well as providing information, advice, and perhaps counselling and carer support. The Parkinson's Disease Society, or similar self-help groups, can also provide useful lay literature, peer support, and a social outlet. Overall, treatment and rehabilitation should, if possible, be community focused and away from the hospital out-patient department where there are limitations on time and access to the multidisciplinary team.

Dystonia

The dystonic syndromes are characterized by sustained involuntary muscle contractions resulting in abnormal movements and postures. There are a variety of presentations from more generalized forms in childhood to the commoner focal dystonias starting in middle life. The commoner sites involved in focal dystonia are the eye (blepharospasm), neck (spasmodic torticollis), jaw, tongue and mouth (oromandibular dystonia), larynx and vocal cords (spasmodic dysphonia), and arm and hand muscles (writer's cramp). Various other segmental, multifocal, and hemidystonic forms also occur.

The majority of dystonias are idiopathic in origin, although recently a genetic tendency has been noted, usually a dominant form of inheritance with reduced penetrance. An accurate diagnosis is necessary in order that secondary dystonias can be appropriately treated. Secondary causes include drug-induced dystonia (particularly psychotropics), rarer yet treatable diseases such as Wilson's disease, cerebral tumours, or arterio-venous malformations. Untreatable causes are sometimes found including the various metabolic disorders of childhood. Diagnosis is still important, particularly from the point of view of discussion of natural history and genetics.

Recent studies have indicated a prevalence of around 15 per 100 000 population, which is commoner than motor neuron disease. There is now a very effective treatment, particularly for focal dystonia, which has had the effect of bringing together individuals with dystonia into defined clinics which in turn as highlighted the need for a multidisciplinary approach.

Treatment

Until recently there was very little satisfactory treatment for any form of dystonia. A variety of drug interventions, particularly anti-cholinergics, have been tried with little success, and often individuals had to resort to heroic surgical interventions, including stereotactic operations and various forms of peripheral denervation. Although a few individuals may still need to resort to such procedures the majority are now treated with the use of botulinum toxin. Botulinum toxin is a potent neurotoxin that inhibits the release of acetyl choline from the nerve endings. The technique simply requires the injection of the toxin into the affected muscle. The muscle slowly relaxes over a 2–3 day period and the effect lasts 2–3 months. Published studies indicate an efficacy of approximately 90 per cent for focal dystonia. Generalized and other forms of dystonia can often be helped by injection in the most affected muscles to produce at least some benefit.

Although the disability is mild in dystonia the handicap can often be severe, and many individuals suffer severe social embarrassment, social isolation, and lost employment as a result of the often bizarre movements.

The advent of botulinum clinics has enabled such individuals to gather together in larger numbers than was the case previously and from such clinics peer-support groups and counselling services can be developed. Recent initiatives such as the use of nurse practitioners to administer botulinum toxin to the patient in their home are now producing further benefit for individuals with this distressing condition.

Huntington's chorea

Huntington's disease is a rare condition with a prevalence in the UK of around 2–10 per 100 000. It is mentioned in this textbook because of the clear requirement for a co-ordinated multidisciplinary approach including neurologists, neuropsychiatrists, therapists, and genetic specialists.

It is a degenerative disorder in which neuronal loss occurs, in the caudate nucleus and putamen, and has a characteristic finding of atrophy of the head of the caudate nucleus on CT scanning. Peak age of onset is around 40 years, which unfortunately means that the individual is often married with a young family and thus with a high chance of having passed the genetic defect on to offspring. It is an autosomal dominant condition with full penetrance so that each offspring with an affected parent has a 1 in 2 risk of contracting the disease. Time from diagnosis to death is in the order of 10–15 years.

The disease itself has a characteristic spectrum of motor, psychiatric, and cognitive problems. Involuntary movements mainly include chorea but can include a variety of other movements including dystonia. Gait is often unsteady and dyspraxic and dysarthria and swallowing problems are also common. Parkinsonian features can dominate, particularly in more juvenile forms of the disorder. Psychiatric disorders are almost universal and can be the presenting feature. Symptoms can vary from apathy to irritability and verbal and physical aggression with a variety of sexual problems, particularly excessive and often inappropriate sexual interest. Clearly major depression is a common feature in a condition in which insight is often preserved for some time. Eventually dementia will dominate, often following a long period of decline in intellectual function, particularly memory impairment. In late stages dementia and profound involuntary movements will predominate.

Genetics

The Huntington's genes are on chromosome 4. Predictive DNA testing is now possible both for the adult who is concerned about inheritance and prenatally in order to assess the risk for the foetus. The reading list points to further literature on this subject. Involvement of a geneticist in the rehabilitation team is now vital.

Treatment

Although the disease is not curable a rehabilitation team can produce invaluable assistance and support. Physiotherapy can often improve gait and can certainly reduce unnecessary physical complications such as contractures. An occupational therapist can likewise assist with activities of daily living and planning of the home and work environments. A speech and language therapist can be very useful for the management of dysphagia. A dietician is often useful because of the significantly increased calorific demands in someone with constant movements. Neuropsychology or neuropsychiatric assessment and intervention can assist with the depressive features and behavioural strategies can be useful to alleviate such problems as aggression and sexual disinhibition.

There are now a number of dedicated units managing people with Huntington's chorea. This trend is to be encouraged given the complexity of the disorder and of rehabilitation management.

Further reading

Agid, Y. (1992). *Current trends in the treatment of Parkinson's disease.* Libbey, London.

Battistin, L., Scarlato, G., Caracen, T., and Ruggieri, S. (1996). *Advances in neurology 69: Parkinson's disease.* Lippincott-Raven, Philadelphia.

Butler, A., Duffey, P., Hawthorne, M., and Barnes, M. (1998). The socio-economic implications of dystonia. *Advances in Neurology 1998; Dystonia*, **3**, (78), 349–58.

Duffey, P., Butler, A. G., Hawthorne, M. R., and Barnes, M. P. (1998). The epidemiology of primary dystonia in the north of England. *Advances in Neurology 1998; Dystonia*, **3**, (78), 121–5.

Harper, P. S. (1991). *Huntington's disease*. Saunders, London.

Kurlan, R. (1995). *Treatment of movement disorders*. Lippincott, Philadelphia.

Marsden, C. D. and Fahn, S. (1994). *Movement Disorders 3*. Butterworth, London.

Raven, N. G., Peyser, C. E., and Folstein, S. E. (1993). *A physicians guide to the management of Huntington's disease: pharmacologic and non-pharmacologic interventions*. Huntington's Disease Society of America, New York.

22

....

Other neurological disabling conditions

It is not the aim of this book to cover all neurological disabling conditions. Rehabilitation medicine focuses on the management of disability and handicap. Most neurological conditions will be managed by the basic principles of rehabilitation combined with the management of specific disabilities, as outlined in other chapters. However, the conditions described in this chapter provide specific challenges to the rehabilitation team and thus are worth discussing in their own right. Details of the aetiology, pathophysiology, and diagnosis will not be covered and the reader is referred to standard neurological textbooks for these issues. The disorders covered in this chapter are motor neuron disease, epilepsy, Guillain–Barré syndrome, and dementia. A brief mention will also be made of polio and the post-polio syndrome as this is the commonest neurological disabling condition world-wide, albeit uncommon in the UK.

Motor neuron disease

Motor neuron disease (MND) is not common but nevertheless provides significant challenges to the rehabilitation team.

Classification, natural history and epidemiology

The prevalence of MND in the UK is around 5 per 100 000 within an incidence of approximately 1 per 100 000 per annum. Thus, the disorder is unusual and normally outside the experience of the general practitioner. The complex range of disabilities requires the input of a specialized rehabilitation team. The disorder is rare before the age of 40 and there is a rising incidence with age thereafter. Men are affected approximately 1.5 times as frequently as women. Family history is unusual but is reported in around 7–10 per cent of cases.

There are a number of forms of the disorder. Amyotrophic lateral sclerosis (ALS) is the commonest type, occurring in about 80 per cent of people. There is a mixture of upper and lower motor neuron problems that give rise to a characteristic range of signs including spasticity, increased reflexes, and muscle weakness in combination with muscle wasting and muscle fasciculation. In this form survival time from diagnosis to death is approximately three years.

Progressive bulbar palsy refers to the variant of the condition involving the bulbar muscles, usually both the lower and upper motor neurons. This gives rise to distressing and dangerous problems such as dribbling, dysarthria, dysphagia, and respiratory infection. This variant has the worse prognosis with a median survival of 2–3 years.

Progressive muscular atrophy is a rarer form involving only the lower motor neurons of the limbs and having a better survival with a median time of more than five years. Primary lateral sclerosis is a very rare pure upper motor neuron form of the disorder.

Another form of the disorder is lathyrism which gives rise to spastic paraparesis and is caused by eating the pea vetch *Lathyrus sativus*. This disease is endemic in Bangladesh, India, Ethiopia, and other developing countries, particularly at times of famine. A final type which is common in some Western Pacific islands (Guam and Rota in the Marianas) is thought to be due to eating flour made from the ripe seeds of cycascircanalis. This form of the disorder is associated with Parkinsonism and dementia.

Giving the diagnosis

In the vast majority of cases motor neuron disease progresses inexorably to death within a few years. Proper information and support from the time of diagnosis is vital. Once the diagnosis has been confirmed the individual and main partner or close family members should be given time to hear about the likely course of the disease and the possible management of the various disabilities and more particularly the support that can, and cannot, be offered for the various symptoms. It is often important to allow the individual and family to return for a second consultation after further thoughts and questions have arisen. Literature written in clear lay language should be available and the name and address of the Motor Neurone Disease Association should be given. The Association can supply literature, peer support, and counselling. In most parts of the UK there is a regional advisor of the MNDA who can visit people at home and can often provide practical support such as loan of equipment as well as emotional support to the family. The individuals should certainly keep in touch with the rehabilitation team in order that treatment interventions can be initiated before unnecessary complications arise.

Medical treatment

The history of MND is littered with a variety of unsuccessful therapies. There is some evidence that the use of branch chain amino acids can slow down the disease process. However, at the present time there is no convincing treatment intervention.

Major problems and rehabilitation management

Mobility and activities of daily living

A major problem for the individual is increasing weakness of both arms and legs due to the combination of upper and lower motor neuron dysfunction. Advice on gait and passive exercises to reduce the risk of contractures are important in the early stages. Eventually it is likely that a

wheelchair will be required. Often the seating requirements are complicated by the need for trunk, neck, and
head support. Although sensation is preserved there is a
still a significant risk of pressure sores from immobility and
proper attention needs to be paid to cushioning requirements. Whilst there is still functional movement of the arms
a variety of simple aids to daily living can be useful and
advice sought from an occupational therapist and/or a
disabled living centre.

Respiratory and bulbar problems

The main disability and indeed the most distressing
problems arise from bulbar involvement. Most individuals
will experience dysphagia, dribbling, choking, dysarthria,
and communication problems as well as respiratory weakness at some point. Dysphagia arises from muscle weakness
and problems of coordination of the tongue and swallowing mechanism. An assessment by a speech and language
therapist, often involving videofluroscopy, is necessary in
order to give valid advice. Usually feeding will become slow
and tiring and it may be preferable to use a percutaneous
endoscopic gastrostomy sooner rather than later. This will
maintain calorie intake and reduce, but not remove, the risk
of aspiration and malnutrition.

In the short term a speech therapist might be able to
assist with the problems of dysarthria and dysphonia but
often individuals will need to resort to a communication
aid. There are a number of devices on the market which
allow even the most severely disabled person to communicate effectively.

Respiratory failure

Involvement of the respiratory muscles of the neck and
intercostals as well as phrenic nerve damage can all
seriously compromise respiration. There is always the
additional risk of aspiration. Advice from a physiotherapist
regarding chest drainage, intermittent suction, and positioning is important. Portable suction devices should be
available as and when necessary within the home. There
may come a point when ventilatory assistance is required.
However, in the later stage ethical questions will arise as to

whether artificial ventilation is justified. There can be no rigid guidelines and such decisions will need to be taken in close conjunction with the individual and family.

Late stages and death
Insight into the condition normally remains and consequently there is a high incidence of depression. This should be recognized and as far as possible treated, preferably by cognitive therapy and not by sedative anti-depressant medication.

Most studies have demonstrated that individuals prefer to stay at home during their terminal stage. This will often require complex, albeit short-term, care packages involving experienced nurses and with the support of the physician and physiotherapist and a dietician for respiratory and nutritional management. Death is normally from bronchopneumonia. Doses of morphine and/or prochlorperazine and hyoscine can be used to relieve distress and diminish bronchial secretion. Difficult ethical questions are now being publicly debated regarding assisted suicide. In most countries this is still illegal but it is worth pointing out that a physician has no ethical, legal, or moral obligation to prolong the distress of a dying individual.

Polio

Polio is now extremely uncommon in developed countries and becoming rapidly less common in the developing world following an intensive immunization campaign by the WHO. However, the physical consequences of polio are still amongst the commonest disabling disorders in less developed countries and post-polio syndrome is still quite common world-wide. In most new cases polio is not accompanied by any symptoms only by mild systemic flu-like symptoms or gastroenteritis. In a small proportion of people there is a mild attack of aseptic meningitis. Only in a very tiny number does a paralytic polio myelitis syndrome arise. In these cases muscle weakness develops rapidly over 48 hours. The distribution of paralysis is variable ranging from focal paralysis in a single limb to a more widespread symmetrical paralysis reminiscent of Guillain–Barré syndrome. Bulbar muscle involvement is more common in young adults. Survival is threatened if there is involvement of the respiratory musculature and/or phrenic nerve. The overall mortality rate of acute paralytic polio is around 5–10 per cent. Most people recover completely over 3–4 months. In a small proportion (possibly around 10 per cent) there is residual disability which is usually confined to the legs. The flaccid paralysis can usually be assisted by correct use of orthoses and/or special shoes and a variety of walking aids. Rarely surgery is required in order to improve functional ability by such procedures as tendon transfers.

Post-polio syndrome occurs at least 15 years after the original attack. After recovery there is a period of stabilization and then very slowly new difficulties begin such as increasing weakness, further loss of muscle bulk, and fatigue with consequent decreased functional ability. These symptoms are usually observed in muscles that have been previously affected. Post-polio syndrome is slowly progressive and treatment will focus on methods to assist weak limbs, particularly the use of orthoses, mobility aids, and wheelchairs.

Guillain–Barré syndrome

Acute inflammatory polyneuropathy (Guillain–Barré syndrome) affects children and adults of all ages. Although the cause is unknown it is usually preceded by a mild respiratory or gastrointestinal infection. The incidence is approximately 1 per 100 000 population per annum. Limb weakness usually evolves more or less symmetrically over a period ranging from a few days to 1–2 weeks. Weakness usually spreads from distal to more proximal muscles involving both the upper and lower extremities, usually the legs first. Eventually the trunk, intercostal, neck, and cranial nerves can all be involved. Occasionally motor progress is rapid from initial stages to motor paralysis and death from respiratory failure within a day or so. Objective sensory loss and paraesthesiae can occur to a variable degree. The mortality rate is around 5 per cent. In the short term the most important requirement is respiratory support as well as appropriate care of the consequences of immobility including bladder and bowel management, passive movement of the limbs and avoidance of pressure sores. The majority of individuals recover over several months but a significant minority (around 15–20 per cent) will have residual disabilities. Treatment, as for polio, usually needs to be directed towards weak limbs with the use of orthoses, walking aids, wheelchairs, and car modifications as necessary. Very rarely long-term respiratory support is required and occasionally there is a long-term bulbar involvement requiring, for example, percutaneous endoscopic gastrostomy feeding and augmentative communication aids. The only useful medical treatment is plasmapharesis with plasma exchange taking place as rapidly as possible after the onset of the disorder. Steroids are sometimes used early but are of doubtful efficacy. Intravenous immunoglobulin has also been used and may provide modest benefit.

Epilepsy

Epilepsy is remarkably common. It has been estimated that between 2 and 5 per cent of the entire population will suffer at least one non-febrile seizure during their lives. The overall prevalence is around 5000 per 100 000 with an incidence of around 50 per 100 000 per annum. It is thus the single most common disabling neurological condition in both adults and children. It is not a condition that is often seen by a multidisciplinary rehabilitation team due to the inherent intermittent nature of the condition and lack of disability between attacks. However, the rehabilitation team is increasingly recognized as necessary for psychosocial support.

Medical management

This chapter will not deal with the classification of epilepsy nor with the details of pharmacological management. An accurate diagnosis is essential as is adequate discussion about the natural history, prognosis, and potential treatment. Diagnosis is not always clear from the history and examination, and periods of in-patient observation using EEG telemetry and television monitoring may be needed. There is now a wide choice of drugs. The great majority of individuals can be adequately controlled on a single anti-convulsant, although a small number will require multiple therapy. The longer-standing drugs include phenytoin, sodium valproate, and carbamazepine and are still the most widely used. Phenobarbitone is still used globally because it is cheap and effective, albeit with an unsatisfactory range of side effects. In the last few years a number of new anti-convulsants have become available including lamotrigine, gabapentine, vigabatrin, topiramate, and others. These new compounds are mainly used as second-line treatment at the moment although are beginning to find a place as first-line options.

Unfortunately many people are lost to follow-up after initial stabilization on an anti-convulsant regime. Limited follow-up is acceptable for some people with infrequent seizures who are well controlled on a stable anti-convulsant regime but it is recommended that everyone with epilepsy should be reviewed intermittently. Only about 6 per cent of people attend a dedicated epilepsy clinic. It has been found that those who do attend such clinics are given and retain more information about their epilepsy and are more satisfied with the service received and support given than those attending routine neurological or other medical clinics. A dedicated epilepsy service should involve other professionals, including nursing staff trained in epilepsy management and psychological and counselling support as well as support from local epilepsy groups.

Neuropsychological assessment and support

Most people with epilepsy have well controlled seizures with no significant cognitive problems. However, those with frequent or poorly controlled seizures are at risk of cognitive deficits. This is a result of the epilepsy itself, another underlying disorder, or as a consequence of anti-convulsant medication. Memory problems are the commonest of these deficits. There are now a wide range of appropriate strategies that can help cope with memory difficulties (see Chapter 16). Neuropsychological assessment can be used to monitor an individual's cognitive performance both before and after drug changes, and the psychologist may thus advise when the drug is having a deleterious impact on cognitive functioning, including information-processing speed, memory, and concentration. Such changes can improve on withdrawal of medication or reduction of dosage. Clinical anxiety or depression can occur. Anxiety can itself trigger seizures and produce further anxiety and is thus best treated actively. Relaxation therapy has been shown to produce a significant reduction in seizure frequency in individuals prone to clinical anxiety. Depression is probably best managed by cognitive strategies rather than anti-depressant medication although the latter is sometimes required. Aggression can also occur in epilepsy, sometimes as part of the epileptic event. It can also arise during periods of postictal confusion.

Social aspects of epilepsy

The diagnosis of epilepsy can have a profound effect on social life and cause significant handicap. There is a much higher level of unemployment in people with epilepsy. A trained epilepsy worker, often a social worker or nurse, should help with job applications and should visit the employer to explain the nature of the disorder. Counselling for the individual may be required as some have unrealistic expectations of employment and fail to perceive the health and safety issues that arise for an employer. Some occupations will clearly be out of the question including flying, commercial diving, operating hazardous machinery, working at heights, and public service vehicle and commercial driving. A detailed appraisal of the type and frequency of fit and of the job itself may be required and close liaison maintained with the employment rehabilitation service. Restrictions on driving can also place people with epilepsy at a disadvantage. Recent changes in the UK driving legislation allow people to drive as long as there has been a seizure-free period of at least one year, or attacks have only occurred whilst asleep for a period of at least three years. The onus of responsibility for informing the Driver and Vehicle and Licensing Agency (DVLA) in Swansea rests with the licence holder and not the physician. This is not the case in all countries.

The family of the person with epilepsy will often need to be involved with the rehabilitation process. The family's attitude to epilepsy and their understanding of the nature of the disorder is important. In particular support and guidance will need to be given to children, particularly the first-aid management of a parent or sibling with epilepsy. In children with epilepsy there is often a difficult balance to be maintained between normal risk-taking behaviour and over-protection resulting in potential psychological problems.

Finally, at all ages there is clear evidence that epilepsy can lead to social isolation. Guidance may need to be given on pursuit of active but appropriate leisure interests, social pursuits, management of relationships, education and further education, and employment.

Overall, there is far more to epilepsy than the management of anti-convulsant medication and there is a clear need for involvement of a expert team in order to minimize disability and handicap.

Dementia

Dementia is not a subject that is usually associated with rehabilitation. The diagnosis of dementia is usually a sign for withdrawal of an active rehabilitative process. It is a diagnosis that is not commonly encountered in rehabilitation medicine as such individuals are usually elderly and intervention it is usually by a psychogeriatric team. However, dementia is not that uncommon in the younger population and can be associated with a number of the commoner neurological disabling diseases including Parkinson's disease, stroke, and multiple sclerosis. This brief section does not aim to be comprehensive but will point out a few approaches that may help the dementing person in a rehabilitation environment.

General guidelines

Dementia can pose immense problems. It is, by definition, a global impairment of function including intellectual, memory, other higher cortical functions, perception, language, self-care, and emotional and behavioural control. The first task is a complete multidisciplinary assessment in order to identify the areas of inability as well as the areas of ability. It is important to note the areas of preserved skills and interests that can be used to keep a person in touch with their self and their environment. Reassessment at frequent intervals is also important as dementia is generally a progressive process and areas of preserved function will clearly change over time and different strategies will need to be implemented. Realistic aims will need to be adopted at all times with a general principle of maximizing independence, minimizing dependency, and maintaining quality of life. As most people with dementia are looked after in the community by friends and relatives the need to support carers is also paramount, particularly through practical help at home and periods of respite. By such methods people with dementia can hopefully remain within the community and avoid the indignity and problems associated with residential and nursing home care.

The field of rehabilitation in dementia is under-researched and many treatment approaches have not been properly evaluated. However, the following general approaches have been shown to be helpful, some proven in controlled studies, single case studies, or frankly seem to be simple common sense.

Environmental adaptation

It is often clear that a person with dementia is more stable and functions better in their home or other familiar environment. Cognitive function will often worsen if a person is taken into an unfamiliar hospital ward or different social setting. Thus, the stability of the physical environment is important and in rehabilitation units it is important to achieve a home-like atmosphere and a domestic style of furniture. People should have their own clothes and possessions. This will also imply easy accessibility to washing, toileting, and dining facilities as well as clear directions to such facilities. The latter can be facilitated by clear sign-posting and colour coding.

Stimulation activity

Recently there has been some evaluation of the effects of sensory stimulation including music, touch, taste, and smell. Similar programmes are being proposed for people in persistent coma (see Chapter 20). Results are not clear cut, but it does seem that some forms of sensory input can improve function. It certainly seems clear that absence of sensory stimulation in boring residential environments can compound behavioural disturbance. Sensory stimulation has the added benefit of providing carers with some means of interaction and the appearance of giving some support to the demented relative. Physical activity and general occupation of time through old hobbies and interests are important to provide some stimulus, and perhaps functional benefit.

Reminiscence

Reminiscence therapy utilizes the individual's past memories which, at least in the early stages of dementia, are reasonably intact. Use of the individual's own materials such as photo albums or other published material such as old newspapers and magazines can act as prompts and memory triggers. There is evidence that such techniques increase interaction which can generalize beyond the activity itself. Furthermore the activity has clearly been shown to be enjoyable.

Reality orientation

Reality orientation (RO) has been much discussed in the literature and reasonably evaluated. The aim is to help the person with dementia to continue to experience success and achievement, have increased awareness of present reality, and enhance communication and personal contact. Regular RO sessions up to five times a week lasting about half an hour can show benefit in terms of orientation. There is conflicting evidence whether such techniques produce improvements in behaviour and cognitive functioning, although there is evidence that individuals can find their way round the home more effectively following such sessions. Usually the sessions are conducted in small groups working on activities to increase awareness of surroundings and of those people around them.

Drug management

There has recently been renewed interest in drug therapy for dementias. Most work has focused around the use of cholinergic agents. There is very limited evidence of long-term benefit at the present time. These agents tend to be more widely prescribed in mainland Europe than in the UK and there has been controversy over the costs of such agents compared to their benefits. The exception to this rule is the recent use of Riluzole in an attempt to improve cognitive function. There is some limited evidence that this can be the case and the drug is beginning to be prescribed in some centres. Further studies are necessary to find its exact place in the overall management of Alzheimer's disease. Donepezil and Rivastigmine are centrally acting acetyl cholinesterase inhibitors to prevent the breakdown of central acetyl choline increasing the amount available for synaptic transmission. These drugs do not delay, stop, or cure Alzheimer's dementia but when used in mild to moderate disease they may improve some of the early symptoms.

Behavioural management

Behavioural management techniques have been used with some success to increase participation in social activities and reduce the amount of inappropriate social behaviour such as shouting or sexual disinhibition. This subject is discussed in more detail in Chapter 13. It is important to involve the family and carers and to make them, as far as possible, the vehicles for change and ongoing contact. This can help to reduce the sense of nihilism that can occur in relentlessly progressive conditions.

Further reading

Motor neuron disease

Cochrane, G. M. (ed.) (1987). *The management of motor neurone disease*. Churchill Livingstone, London.

Cochrane, G. M. and Donaghy, M. (1993). Motor neuron disease. In: Greenwood, R., Barnes, M. P., McMillan, T. M., and Ward, C. D. (ed.) *Neurological rehabilitation*, pp.571–87. Churchill Livingstone, London.

Williams, A. C. (1994). *Motor neuron disease*. Chapman and Hall Medical, London.

Polio

Gourie-Devi, M. (1996). Poliomyelitis and other anterior horn cell disorders. In: Shakir, R. A., Newman, P. K., and Poser, C. M. (ed.) *Tropical neurology*, pp.95–121. Saunders, London.

Smith, L. K. and Mabry, M. (1995). Poliomyelitis and the postpolio syndrome. In: Umphred, D. A. (ed.) *Neurological rehabilitation*, pp.571–87. Mosby, St Louis, MO.

Guillain Barré Syndrome

Hickey, J. V. (1992). Guillain Barré syndrome. In: Hickey, J. V. (ed.) *Neurological and neurosurgical nursing*, pp.651–6. Lippincott, Philadelphia.

Epilepsy

Engel, J. and Pedley, T. A. (1997). *Epilepsy. A comprehensive textbook*, Vols. 1, 2, and 3. Lippincott-Raven, Philadelphia.

Dementia

Woods, R. T. (1993). Rehabilitation of Alzheimer's disease and other dementias. In: Greenwood, R., Barnes, M. P., McMillan, T. M., and Ward, C. D. (ed.) *Neurological rehabilitation*, pp.517–24. Churchill Livingstone, London.

23

....

Arthritis

Arthritis is the largest cause of locomotor disability in developed countries. While management of patients with arthritis is usually the responsibility of rheumatologists and orthopaedic surgeons, there are many features in which a rehabilitationist becomes involved. Patients with mobility problems may require therapy. a wheelchair, or an orthosis and those with severe disabilities may require the help of a multiprofessional team, especially if they develop complications. Examples of the latter include the development of cervical myelopathy in severe rheumatoid arthritis or spondylosis/spondylitis. The resources of most rheumatology services are insufficient to provide the necessary help for all the patient's needs and a rehabilitationist's input may be useful. It is therefore important to have a detailed knowledge of these diseases and rheumatological/locomotor rehabilitation is thus included in the curriculum for higher specialist training in rehabilitation medicine. This chapter will now describe some of the main arthritides: rheumatoid arthritis, sero-negative arthritis, and osteoarthritis.

Rheumatoid arthritis

Rheumatoid arthritis (RA) has an incidence of 30 per 100 000 and a prevalence of 1000 per 100 000, which makes it the most common of the inflammatory arthropathies. Much is now known about the pathophysiology in rheumatoid disease, which presents classically as a symmetrical poly-arthritis affecting small joints with onward progression to involve larger joints. Any joint can be involved and the basic lesion is of a chronic synovitis. Not only can joints suffer inflammation causing pain, swelling, tenderness, and loss of function, but the disease can be systemic and affect a multitude of target organs, some of which are shown in table 23.1.

Despite the considerable advances in disease modification over the last 20 years, rheumatoid arthritis still causes a

Table 23.1   Extra-articular manifestations of rheumatoid disease

Affected organ	Manifestation
Eyes	Sjogren's syndrome, keratoconjunctivitis sicca, scleritis
Heart	Pericarditis, myocarditis, valve abnormalities, Raynaud's phenomenon
Lungs	Alveolitis, pleural effusions, nodules, blood vessels, vasculitis producing micro-infacts, rashes, neuropahty, ulcers etc. Crico-arytenoid joint arthritis
Skin	Rash, ulcers, nerves, vasculitis lesions
Nervous system	Compression syndromes, sensory-mtoor neuropathies, encephalomyelitis
Spinal cord	Transverse myelitis, cord compression
Gut	Dysphagia from Sjogren's syndrome, bowel infarcts (drug-induced gastro-intestinal problems)
Kidneys	Glomerulonephritis, immune complex disease, amyloidosis
Blood	Anaemia of chronic inflammation, Felty's syndrome, thrombocytosis
Reticulo-endothegial system	Lymphadenopathy, Felty's syndrome, non-specific hepatitis
General	Nodule formation, particularly in subcutaneous tissues over areas of pressure

significant disability for many sufferers. The impact of the disease in respect of mobility, the need for care at home, work attendance, and health care expenditure is considerable, and reliance on health care professionals persists. While life and quality of life can be prolonged, active rehabilitation is required to improve abilities and function, better attendance at work, and a better outlook of life. Furthermore, prevention of the complications and joint protection are vital elements in this process.

Natural history

The distribution of rheumatoid arthritis is quite different from that of osteoarthritis and the chronic synovitis proceeds to form a pannus, causing joint destruction. The pathognomic feature is the presence of erosions of articular cartilage and its underlying bone. Untreated, this leads to joint destruction, instability, and loss of function. There is a florid synovitis in rheumatoid disease which further destroys cartilage and bone and leads to overall disruption of the joint. Many joints can be affected and symptoms present due to loss of overall function of that particular part and to pain and stiffness. Because of pain inhibition and general ill-health, muscles supporting the joints become wasted and lose function, thereby causing further disability. Rheumatoid disease therefore has a major impact on mobility and dexterity, as well as on general health. Those patients with a positive rheumatoid factor, which is a circulating IgM immunoglobulin are termed as seropositive and tend to have more aggressive disease (although this is not always the case), but 15 per cent of patients have a seronegative rheumatoid arthritis. Compromise to the patient's health is usually caused by the non-articular complications of the disease. Treatment is aimed at limiting the effects of the disease, for, as yet, there is no cure for this condition. Disease modification has certainly been much more successful over recent years and new agents have been found, which have been used with great skill. One now sees far less of the terrible joint destruction that used to occur, giving rise to deformities and disability. There is also a possibility that over this century rheumatoid disease has become less severe, as improvements have occurred in the general health and living conditions of that population. The natural history of the disease is to burn itself out after 10 to 20 years. The residual disability at the end of this time depends on the degree of joint destruction and musculo-skeletal deformity. Certainly, a proportion of the patients have physical disabilities which require rehabilitation and help, but the majority function fairly independently. The difficulty in rheumatoid arthritis is that, once the rheumatoid process becomes quiescent, the patient is still left with joint destruction and secondary osteoarthritis and may have permanent damage to other target organs.

Surgery has a significant role in rheumatoid disease and a special group of interested orthopaedic surgeons has been formed to promote good practice in the surgery of rheumatoid patients. It is very important that before any surgery is contemplated, the overall aims of treatment and expected outcomes are explained to the patient and his or her family. Anaesthetists should also take note of the vulnerability of the cervical spine in patients with rheumatoid disease and all patients going to the operating theatre should wear a cervical collar, not so much as a protective device, but as a reminder for the theatre staff.

Surgery is most effective during an inactive phase of the disease and possibly after the disease has burnt itself out. Procedures in the hand may improve function and one of the classic indications for surgery is the rupture of the fourth and fifth extensor tendons, as they pass over the ulnar styloid at the wrist. The intense synovitis in the wrist causes a triggering feeling and eventually rupture of the extensor tendons as they pass over the bony prominence. Urgent treatment is required, as even a short delay of a few days may result in an inability to repair the tendons successfully. The patient notices over a short time an inability to extend the fourth and fifth fingers. If tendon surgery is not effective, a lively splint may have to be worn to overcome the disability.

Synovectomy used to be a common operation in rheumatoid disease, but is now much less often performed. The aim was to debulk some of the synovial thickening in the joint and thus to reduce the pain and loss of function in the joint. However, it often gave rise to marked stiffness and has been superceded by more effective medical management. Similarly, arthrodesis used to be a common procedure to fuse the joint and thus reduce pain. In this respect, it was highly effective in its aims, but has now been superceded by joint replacement, particularly in the hips and knees. The resultant disability caused by an arthrodesed knee is quite significant, particularly in the presence of other joint disease. Hip, knee, and shoulder arthroplasties have become very effective, and the first two are now commonly carried out. Elbow replacement is becoming increasingly possible, but is still at a relatively early stage in its development. The ankle joint is a difficult joint to replace and the effects of ankle arthrodesis are so much better at the present time. Although it gives rise to a stiff ankle, it is successful in relieving pain at the joint. Most people can cope quite well with the resultant impairment and arthroplasty does not seem to confer much added benefit at the present time. Finally, there are a whole host of other operative procedures, such as carpal tunnel decompression, as this condition is more common in rheumatoid patients. Surgery to the spine, and in particular to the lower part of the neck, may have to be considered where cervical myelopathy is a danger, and fusion of the cervical spine may be required at both the atlanto-occipital and atlanto-axial levels and in the lower cervical spine.

Important issues in the rehabilitation of patients with RA

So what do we need to know about rheumatoid patients prior to setting up a rehabilitation programme? Obviously, it is vital to get a comprehensive history and to examine the patient fully. Rather than just document painful and swollen joints, there are specific issues which will have an impact on the life of the patient and on his or her rehabilitation. These include:
- Fatigue
- Joint pain and stiffness
- Skeletal deformities
- Soft tissue swelling
- Mobility and daily activity

....

- Psychosocial problems
- Environmental issues.

Rheumatoid disease is a progressive condition and while an assessment early on in the disease may produce a certain set of findings, certain features can herald a deterioration. In this respect, it is important to know the functional performance and the capacity for further improvement in performance. It is also necessary to know which features of the disease are reversible and which are not and to learn which activities are tolerated and which are not.

Diurnal variations in performance are obviously important, and early morning stiffness is not only a marker of disease activity, but has an impact on the patient's lifestyle. Underpinning the rehabilitation process is the need for effective medication and rheumatologists have become much more proactive in starting second-line or disease-modifying agents. The side effects are better controlled, patients are better monitored, and these potentially harmful drugs are better tolerated in skilled hands. Non-steroidal anti-inflammatory drugs (NSAIDs) may reduce pain and stiffness, but do not modify the disease process and are therefore used for symptomatic relief only. They too have side effects, of which one of the most common is gastro-intestinal upset.

Management

Rehabilitation is involved at all levels and the process must continually be reappraised by the attending physician, but essentially management falls into three main areas:
- Control of pain and physical treatment
- Anti-arthritic drug treatment
- Protection and preservation of function.

Control of pain and physical treatment
The importance of physical treatment in the management of all joint disease cannot be underestimated. The diagnosis of rheumatoid arthritis still carries a pessimistic outlook in the view of the general public and much support is needed. This can be given by all members of the treating team and the main aim of such treatment is to reduce pain.

It is important to deal with the pain of rheumatoid disease, which may be of two types: acute joint flares, which are severe and debilitating, but whose treatment is likely to resolve fairly rapidly, and the chronic underlying pain of rheumatoid disease, which affects the joints, muscles, and limbs and leads to significant disability. Many patients become quite depressed and exhausted, which increases the impact of their pain. Rehabilitation must control pain, promote normalization of responses and maintain lifestyle to as great a degree as possible. Preservation of sleep is a prime factor, which allows patients to face the next day in better shape.

Physical treatment for relief of pain includes cold, heat, electricity, water, and light, such as laser treatment. Transcutaneous nerve stimulation and acupuncture are also widely used, along with exercise, both on dry land and in water. Cold packs have been found to be good analgesics, as effective as heat in increasing the range of shoulder movement in adhesive capsulitis. Cold packs should be applied for about 10 min to swollen, stiff, and painful joints, and pain reduction occurs through reduction of muscle spasm. Care must be taken not to precipitate an exacerbation of Raynaud's phenomenon, which may occur even after only 10 min of application.

Heat may be administered in various ways and hot packs are very useful in muscle aching and stiffness. Hand stiffness can be helped by immersion in warm wax baths and the main indication is for subacute joint pain and for stiffness. It should not really be used in acute situations as it may increase the metabolic rate and thus the degree of inflammation. Hydrotherapy also delivers heat and is very useful in mobilizing stiff joints. The exercise effect can also have benefits on sleep and provides analgesia over short periods of time. Ultrasound delivers heat and can penetrate skin to a depth of about 5 cm. It is also therefore a reasonably good analgesic and can increase the distensibility of tissue. While so many modalities appear to be effective in a whole range of conditions, physiotherapy treatments in general require more comprehensive studies of effectiveness.

Electric treatment reduces pain and muscle spasm in rheumatoid disease. While low intensity laser treatment is widely used, it has not been shown to be any more effective than any other therapy in a whole range of conditions and a question mark perhaps stands over its clinical value. Fortunately, it does not appear to be at all harmful.

Two forms of treatment which have become increasingly useful are transcutaneous electrical nerve stimulation (TENS or TNS) and acupuncture. The former delivers small stimuli to sensory nerves, which block depolarization at the dorsal root entry zone in the spinal cord and 'close the gate' to further stimuli from a painful source. Sensory input is maintained, but the patient feels less pain while the stimulus is applied. There is in addition some carry-over after the stimulator has been turned off and this allows patients to manage the pain throughout a 24 hour period. It can be applied in a whole host of conditions and can deal with both local and referred pain. Electrodes are applied to the skin over the painful area or even at distant areas along acupuncture meridians. It tends to be more effective when applied locally and can result in reducing the amount of analgesia the patient requires. Certainly it has good reports and studies show it to be effective. Acupuncture has been an adjunct to pain relief in a variety of conditions for thousands of years. Several studies have now reported its efficacy for the relief of joint pain in rheumatoid disease and there is a possibility that it may influence cellular and humeral responses in rheumatoid disease. There is scope for this treatment in the future, but it should be carried out by a proficient acupuncturist.

Orthoses
One of the best ways to settle an acute joint flare is to rest that part of the limb. Bedrest may be necessary, but is becoming less acceptable in view of complications. Splinting of joints may be useful in gaining local relief, not only of the structures within the joint, but of the surrounding soft tissues as well. Combining the skills of doctors, occupational therapists, physiotherapists, podiatrists, and orthotists can ensure clear aims of treatment to protect joints and limbs as much as possible. Orthoses have been described in greater detail in Chapter 13, but essentially they either immobilize body parts in functional positions or

substitute for lost function. Both static and dynamic splints have their individual uses, but it is useful in the context of rheumatoid disease to identify some of the key issues. The hand has four main functions which need to be addressed when considering an orthosis. These are the power grip, when the wrist is slightly extended and when the fingers are flexed at the metacarpo-phalangeal and interphalangeal joints, the pinchgrip, when the thumb and index finger are in contact, the key grip, when there is opposition of the thumb to the side of the index finger, and the hook grip, which, for instance allows a suitcase or handbag to be carried on flexed MCP and IP joints. The wrist is in a neutral position and the thumb is not involved in the latter function.

Lower limb orthoses are used primarily for immobilization and for support. One of the important features in rheumatoid disease is the potential to develop subtalar valgus subluxation and subsequent deformity. This in itself produces mid-foot and forefoot pain and pronates the foot. The consequence of this is to compress the lateral plantar nerve, as it passes under the arch of the foot between it and the quadratus plantae muscle, causing pain and numbness in the lateral aspect of the foot. As the condition progresses, foot pronation increases and the medial plantar nerve also becomes stretched on leaving the tarsal tunnel at the distal end of the flexor retinaculum producing medial foot pain and sensory changes. In severe cases, motor dysfunction can occur in the small muscles of the foot. This is the situation seen in people with sero-positive disease of more than 10 years' duration but it is now known that the wearing of heel insoles to correct subtalar strain from early on after diagnosis can prevent this complication.

Treatment of the foot in both inflammatory and degenerative joint disease can be very difficult and is often overlooked by clinicians. Foot pain can be very disabling and the use of good footwear with and without insoles is important. This is addressed in greater detail in Chapter 12.

The wearing of collars and spinal supports always raises controversy. In rheumatoid arthritis, C1/1 instability must be addressed and prevented. Good posture is necessary, particularly while the patient is asleep. Surgical stabilization of the spine should be considered if there is more then 8 mm of subluxation between the odontoid peg and the atlas, and the wearing of a Halo splint should be considered at about 6 mm. A rigid neck brace with chin support (e.g. a SOMI type brace) is recommended for physical activity in which flexion and extension may occur. Other collars, such as the Philadelphia collar, are also available which is better tolerated because it in fact allows more flexion and extension.

One of the main difficulties with all braces and orthoses is the difficulty in putting them on and taking them off (donning and doffing). Patients with small-joint arthritis of the hands and with osteoarthritis often have considerable trouble with either dexterity or access to the affected part.

Medical treatment

As stated above, medication is increasingly effective in modifying the disease process. Gold and Penicillamine have been used for many years as second-line agents in rheumatoid disease and are effective. More recently, Sulphasalazine and Methotrexate are being used increasingly early on in the disease in order to prevent joint damage and ensure a better overall outcome once the disease burns out. There is a defined group of patients who have a positive anti-nuclear antigen and rheumatoid factor, who express the HLA-D3 gene and who respond very well to hydroxychloroquine. Intra-articular and systemic steroids are also of use in preventing either local or generalized joint flares respectively. They should be accompanied by a period of rest followed by mobilization of the affected part.

Joint protection and education

The most important factor in education of the patient relates to their lifestyle. Listed below are some of the decisions that are required in ensuring that quality of life can be maintained:

1. Is sufficient time given for personal activities of daily living?
2. Are disability aids required for your own personal care or domestic activities?
3 Is help required for personal care or domestic activities?

4. What is your role within the family and among significant others? (has this changed due to the arthritis?)
5. What help is required for you to maintain your employment/occupational activity?
6. What aspects of activities can you ignore or delegate to others?
7. What must be done today, this week, this month, this year?
8. Is time for leisure, recreation and rest incorporated into your daily/weekly plan?
9. What arrangements are being made for significant events, e.g. partnership/marriage, having a family, retirement etc.

The basis of much education is in joint protection and in finding a suitable lifestyle. Clearly, adapting the home and the environment to suit patients' needs is a necessary step and the role of the occupational therapist in this area of work is of primary importance. Help is available from various booklets which are produced by the Arthritis and Rheumatism Council and some are listed in further reading at the end of the chapter.

Outcome measures

Measures of pathology and impairment are well validated and correlated with disease activity. Certainly measuring the acute phase response in the blood give a good indication of the immune response. Disease control correlates with a reduction in the C-reactive protein and in the ESR, but this is not usually adequate for an overall picture of the impact of rheumatoid arthritis. Looking at the impairment gives further information and the Ritchie Articular Index is of use in measuring the pain and tenderness in joints. The sum of the number of joints affected is included in this and other measures include the diameter of joints, which will reduce as joint swelling resolves. The Larsen Score gives an impression of the number of erosions seen on X-ray of selected joints. Again, the hunt for a global score has proved elusive as in many other conditions, and the overall assessment of the disease is made in terms of a combination of pathological markers, impairment scores,

....

and disability and handicap measures. The latter two
domains are more comprehensively covered in Chapter 5
and can be utilized just as easily in arthritis as they can in
neurological disability.

Sero-negative arthritis

Sero-negative arthritis is a term used to describe family of
inflammatory arthritides which include ankylosing spondylitis, Reiter's disease, psoriatis arthritis, post-colitic arthritis
and reactive arthritis. Their main characteristics are involvement of large weight-bearing joints, sacroiliac joints, and
the spine, their relationship to the gastro-intestinal and
genitourinary, ocular, and skin diseases, and the increased
incidence among affected people of the HLA-B27 antigen.
This suggests a genetic linkage between the conditions and
between family members and it is not unknown for different types of sero-negative arthritis to occur in members
of the same family. The discovery of the linkage to the
HLA-B27 antigen is a remarkable story of clinical research.

Characteristics of the disease

Sero-negative arthritis is associated with a 'boggy' synovitis
of large weight-bearing joints, particularly the ankle and
knee. It is also associated with back pain and classically
there is morning stiffness. The pain improves with activity,
but returns along with stiffness with inactivity. Common
features include conjunctivitis, urethritis, colitis, (or in the
case of Crohn's disease any involvement of the gut), and
skin conditions (in particular psoriasis and keratoderma
blenorrhagica). The pain from the arthritis responds to a
greater or lesser extent to non-steroidal anti-inflammatory
drugs, but corticosteroids tend to be unhelpful. The condition usually burns out, but is variable in its length. Sero-
negative arthritis does not usually give rise to major joint
deformities in contrast to rheumatoid disease and the one
constant feature is negativity of the rheumatoid factor.
A treatment plan for sero-negative arthritis is seen in
Table 23.2.

Ankylosing spondylitis (AS)

This is classically an arthritis affecting young men aged 15 to 30. The condition is active for 10 to 20 years. It invariably starts off as a sacroiliitis with low back pain and may proceed to involve the lumbar spine, the thoraco-lumbar junction and the cervical spine. Stiffness is the key symptom along with pain, and the spine may become so stiff that ventilation is reduced. Peripheral joints can also be involved and there can be stiffness of other musculoskeletal structures. In spinal disease, the maintenance of a good truncal position and of hip movements is vital for continued personal functioning. Therefore, regular review is required for measures of chest expansion and lumbar flexion using Schöber's test and a wall to tragus distance. Assessment of lumbar flexion is sometimes carried out by measuring the distance of the finger tips from the ground on forward flexion, but patients with good hip range of movement can give a false impression of lumbar spine stiffness and Schöber's test is much ore reliable. In Schöber's test the patient stands and a mark is made on the back at the level of the iliac crest, i.e. at the level of the L4 vertebral body. Another mark is made 5 cm above this and a third is made 10 cm below. The patient is then asked to touch his toes and the distance between the second and third marks is measured. There should in normal movement be at least a 7 cm difference between standing and bending forward. In the wall to tragus test, one asks the patient to stand against a wall and the distance is simply measured to the tragus of the ear. In addition, sacroiliac joint tenderness is measured by direct palpation and it is also important to measure and document extension and flexion of the hip joints. Preservation of hip extension is the key to maintaining functional mobility in AS. If the hips move normally, one can get by really very well without the need for much alteration in one's lifestyle. Cervical spine movement should also be measured and documented, as advancing disease here can give rise to neurological compression.

The natural consequence of spinal ankylosis in a flexed position is now unusual, but the typical stiff spine may ensue without a programme of regular exercise. It is

Table 23.2 Treatment plan for some sero-negative arthritides

Disease/stage	Treatment
Ankylosing spondylitis	
Early and mild disease	Assessment on review in all cases
	NSAIDs
	Physiotherapy, postural exercises, mobility exercises, breathing exercises, general fitness exercises including swimming.
	Advice about smoking, lifestyle, work, etc.
Moderate disease ± peripheral arthritis	NSAIDs
	Disease modifying drugs will be considered.
	Injection if necessary of selected peripheral joints, exercises as above.
	General measures to address disability and handicap.
Late disease	NSAIDs
	Physio- and occupational therapy for exercises/activities of daily living.
	Address disability and handicap issues.
Psoriatic arthritis	
Mild peripheral disease	Assess and follow-up
	NSAIDs.
	Physiotherapy—muscle strengthening and general fitness exercises.
	Treatment of psoriasis
Progressive peripheral disease	NSAIDs, injection of selected joints, second-line disease-modifying drugs—Salazopryin, Methotrexate.

Treatment of psoriasis
Physiotherapy
Occupational therapy
Surgery to appropriate joints
Address disability & handicap issues

Reiter's disease   Assess and follow-up
NSAIDs
Antibiotic cover for acute attacks
Salazopyrin for persistent disease
Inject appropriate joints and/or enthesopathy
Education on multiple sexual partners and on bowel infection
Physiotherapy
Occupational Therapy
Orthoses if necessary
Surgery if necessary

important that exercise is maintained throughout the course of the disease and smokers must be actively discouraged from continuing their habit. The combination of restricted ventilation and the loss of parenchymal elasticity and ciliary movement caused by smoking comprises a potentially lethal combination.

Psoriatic arthritis

Psoriatic arthritis is a sero-negative arthritis associated with the skin condition psoriasis. Presenting in three forms, it is usually associated with pitting of the nails, which is an indicator that the arthritis is related to the psoriasis. As psoriasis itself is so common, it can occur in combination with sero-positive rheumatoid arthritis and it is important to differentiate between RA and psoriatis arthritis. The three forms of psoriatic arthritis are:
1. A mild peripheral polyarthritis, usually affecting the distal interphalangeal joints, producing pain and stiffness.
2. A severe polyarthritis, causing arthritis mutilans, which is a rapidly progressive, grossly destructive disease and is often associated with florid skin disease. The small joints of the hands are involved and destroyed.
3. A spinal arthritis, closely identified with ankylosing spondylitis. Sacroiliitis occurs, but is not necessarily symmetrical. Clearly, in sacroiliitis, careful examination of the skin is required.

Reiter's disease

This disease classically affects young men and women who are sexually active. It starts with a urethritis or with bowel inflammation. Several days later, a conjunctivitis appears followed by an acute arthritis five to seven days later. The latter can present as unilateral sacroiliitis or more often, as a pauci-articular arthritis affecting one or two large weight-bearing joints. The ankle and knee are typically involved. Classically, also, a plantar fasciitis or other enthesopathy can occur and skin lesions include keratoderma blenorrhagica, which often look like pustular psoriasis. Mucosal lesions occur in the mouth and over the genitals, and in males a circinate balanitis can occur.

The urethritis is often non-specific and can occur after gonococcal urethritis. Treatment should start after investigation to identify an infective agent and *Yersinia, Campylobacter, Shigella,* and *Salmonella* have all been implicated. Initial antibiotic treatment is often recommended along with anti-inflammatories. In persistent cases, the use of Salazopyrin as a disease modifier may also be helpful.

Post-colitic arthritis

Both ulcerative colitis and Crohn's disease are associated with arthritis, which takes on a similar picture to both the peripheral and spinal disease seen in psoriatic arthritis. Again, the peripheral disease usually affects large joints and flares come and go with attacks of bowel disease. Control of the underlying bowel disease usually lease to control of the joint disease and the latter is self-limiting once the gastro-intestinal disease is effectively treated. Colectomy may be required in ulcerative colitis and immunosuppressants in Crohn's disease to achieve this. In contrast, ankylosing spondylitis is independent of any bowel problem, and this condition affects women as commonly as men.

Reactive arthritis

Reactive arthritis or sexually acquired reactive arthritis (SARA) is similar to the above conditions in presentation, but is invariably associated with a non-specific urethritis. It can also occur after non-specific colitis and is a term often used for incomplete features of the above conditions. The response to treatment is similar and the arthritis condition is usually self-limiting. Treatment with antibiotics and anti-inflammatories should be instituted initially and Salazopyrin should also be considered in patients whose symptoms persist.

Osteoarthritis

Despite the fact that degenerative joint disease is common, its incidence is not well known. It is estimated at about 200

per 100 000 population per year for hip and knee osteoarthritis. The prevalence is 3.8 per cent at the knee and
1.3 per cent at the hip, and osteoarthritis is the most
common joint disease in the world. Its impact is therefore
huge.

Definition

The impression of osteoarthritis is that it is due to wear and
tear, but it is not a condition of relentless progression. It is
not actually one disease and represents the endpoint of a
series of insults to the joint. It is not in itself a systemic
disease and its effects are purely local. An imbalance
appears between a joint's ability to withstand stresses and
the actual forces on the joint. Because the joint is continually subjected to new and altered stresses, mild disease
does actually progress to more severe joint failure but this is
a reflection of the endpoint in the underlying process.

Genetic and biochemical factors obviously plays a part
in articular cartilage loss. There is a failure of articular
cartilage matrix which damages its surface and activates
chondrocytes. Repair defects occur resulting in proteo-
glycan loss, collagen damage, and finally cartilage thinning
and loss. Cartilage nutrition is also impaired through a
failure of synovial fluid. Primary and secondary forms are
seen, which are discussed below.

Primary osteoarthritis

This common condition affects women more than men and
is characterized by its distribution through joints and the
presence of Heberden's nodes on the distal interphalangeal
joints. Bouchard's nodes also exist in this condition, but
the osteoarthritis classically affects the knees, hips, distal
interphalangeal joints, the first carpo-metacarpal joint, the
lower cervical spine, and the first metatarso-phalangeal
joint. It occurs in middle-aged and elderly people and is an
annoying but not particularly serious condition. It leads to
pain and swelling in joints and to the need for eventual
joint replacement in hips and knees in more severe cases.
There is an inflammatory condition with a small rise in the

ESR and C-reactive protein. However, the rheumatoid factor is negative and there are no features of rheumatoid disease.

Secondary osteoarthritis

The causes are given in table 23.3. Secondary osteoarthritis can occur as a result of long-standing stresses on a joint. Altered biomechanics from anatomical defects can give rise to forces on a joint over a concentrated area rather than over the whole of the joint surface and the joint will inevitably wear at this point.

Clinical features

The main complaints are pain and stiffness and loss of function due to restricted joint movement and/or instability.

Table 23.3 Causes of secondary osteoarthritis

Cause	Details
Developmental	Anatomical defects resulting in biochemical abnormalities from hyper-mobility syndromes
	Congenital dislocation of hip
	Perthes disease
	Epiphyseal dysplasias
	Infective/septic arthritis
	Inflammation and distant septic focus
	Inflammatory arthritis
	Haemarthrosis etc.
Metabolic	Ochronosis
	Haemochromatosis
	Acromegaly
	Crystal arthritis etc.
Mechanical	Obesity
	Direct trauma
	Previous joint surgery
	Deformity

Patients have diminished standing and walking, and in upper limb disease, decreased dexterity. Sleep is often disturbed and nocturnal pain is a classical feature of the condition. Table 23.4 gives some of the symptoms and signs. Because osteoarthritis does not have systemic effects, the patient's general health is unaffected. Laboratory investigations are normal and clinical features and imaging are the best ways to assess the extent and impact of this disease.

Management

Pain and stiffness should be controlled by analgesia, and acute flares of joint disease may be managed by rest, physiotherapy, and/or local injections of corticosteroids. In chronic pain, anti-depressant drugs may be required to modify the patient's response and supplement analgesics. The European League Against Rheumatism (EULAR) has defined some indications of the impact of medications in osteoarthritis. These are the Index of Severity of Hip and Knee Disease (Lequesne), the investigator's overall opinion, pain on visual analogue scale, patient's global assessment, and walking time. Physical treatment is as for rheumatoid arthritis, but specific issues relate to osteoarthritis. The use of walking sticks and other mobility aids is obviously

Table 23.4   Clinical features of osteoarthritis

Symptoms	Signs
Post-activity stiffness	Joint tenderness
Mild early morning stiffness	Muscle weakness
Pain on activity	Soft tissue swelling around the joint, bony enlargement
Loss of joint function	Joint effusion
Joint swelling	Joint crepitus
Instability	Loss of joint range of movement, instability
Decreased walking speeds	Loss of joint range of movement, instability

important and disability equipment can certainly help osteoarthritic people at home.

Further reading

Butler, R. C. and Jayson, M. I. V. (ed.) (1985–95). *Collected Reports on the Rheumatic Diseases 1985–1995.* (Arthritis and Rheumatism Council)

Klippel, J. H. and Dieppe, P. (1996). *Rheumatology* 2nd edn. Mosby, London.

24
Spinal pain and soft tissue rheumatism

Low back and neck pain are two of the most common conditions encountered by general practitioners, rheumatologists, orthopaedic surgeons, and rehabilitation physicians. The cost of back pain to British industry is 30 to 40 million days annually and approximately 5 per cent of all days off work are due to this cause. The lumbar spine is a complicated structure and pain may result from abnormalities occurring within the bone or the vertebrae, the intervertebral discs, the facet joints, the ligaments, and from the spinal canal and the nerve roots themselves. The spinal cord terminates in the cauda equina at the L1/2 level and below that the canal is packed with spinal nerve roots. In addition to these structures, back pain may be referred from many sites, of which one is from the abdomen, and additionally there may be no structural cause for a person's pain. Psychogenic pain gives rise to back pain among other symptoms.

Back pain

Features: acute syndromes

This will not be considered in much detail, as full accounts will appear in orthopaedic and rheumatological textbooks.

Acute pain may be due to muscular or ligamentous strain, to intervertebral disc prolapse, to facet joint dysfunction, to trauma, or to inflammation or tumours within bone. The treatment of back pain has been described in the CSAG guidelines and bedrest is nowadays not recommended for acute simple low back pain. There is actually no such thing as simple back pain and short-term rest may be useful for some patients in the case of intervertebral disc prolapse, when pain is maybe referred to the leg by nerve root entrapment. When this occurs in a true spinal root distribution, it is known as sciatica, but the term should not be applied to non-spinal root pain referral in the leg and back.

It is important to identify the patient's description of pain. He or she may often refer to buttock pain as hip pain and, unless pinned down, will be quite vague about the distribution of any leg pain. Knowledge of the spine's anatomy (Fig. 24.1) and of the typical radiation patterns of pain are therefore important.

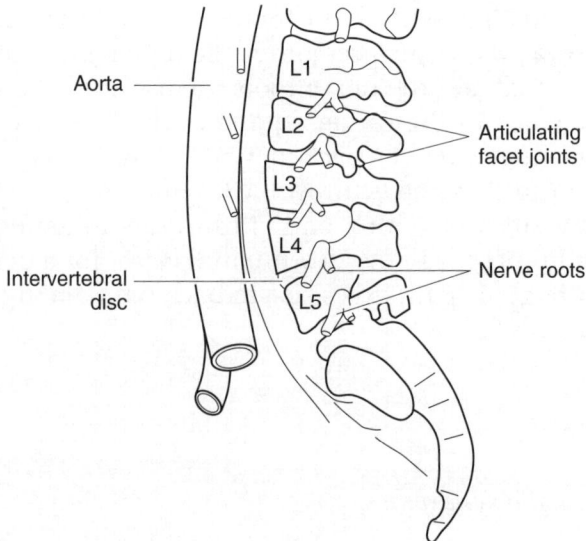

Fig. 24.1 General anatomy of the lumbar spine.

Features: chronic

Many patients have longstanding low back pain. This often starts as an acute pain due to an intervertebral disc prolapse or due to lumbar spondylosis, but chronic pain is characterized more often by features of intermittent acute episodes. These coalesce more and more, such that the patient complains of more constant discomfort. Very often, analgesics are of little help on their own, and the patient requires an explanation of what is going on, as well as a regimen, which he or she can institute at the start of an acute flare of the problem.

Below are some of the more common causes of chronic low back pain, which are further described:

- Posture
- Short leg syndrome
- Degenerative discal disease
- Facet joint pain
- Lumbar spondylosis
- Spondylolisthesis and spondylolysis
- Spinal stenosis
- Diffuse idiopathic skeletal hyperostosis.

Posture

Prolonged poor posture alters the normal curve of the spine and places pressure on the structures therein. Pain is likely to ensue and an enquiry into the person's lifestyle may be helpful. His or her bedding, seating, and activities can all provoke pain, and in particular the position at work or in the car may be worth looking into. Analgesics may be required, but the main priority is to deal with the underlying cause.

Short leg syndrome

Unequal leg lengths will cause tilting of the pelvis. The patient subconsciously adopts a scoliosis in the spine to ensure that the shoulders are symmetrical. This scoliosis will, over a prolonged period of time, cause strain on the ligaments and joints on either side and may cause pain. Correcting the leg length difference with either an insole or shoe raise may be helpful.

....

Prolapsed intervertebral disc

The intervertebral disc is a spacing structure, which in itself probably has no shock-absorbing qualities. It allows the curvature of the spine to occur and is a ring of tough fibrous material—the annulus—which encloses the nucleus pulposus, a gel-like substance, under considerable pressure. On damaging the annulus, extravasation of the nucleus pulposus occurs and pain ensues from the rich neural supply to the closely-applied longitudinal ligament. The onset of sciatica depends on the position of the prolapse and the size of the spinal canal or nerve root foramen. If there is considerable space, back pain alone will occur but if the space is too narrow, then pressure and/or compression on the nerve root will occur, with subsequent leg pain. The lowest intervertebral disc at the L5/L1 level is the most commonly involved, followed by L4/5 and then L3/4. Table 24.1 shows the consequence of disc prolapse at these levels.

Posterolateral protrusions are the most common and affect the nerve root laterally. Posterior or central protrusions are potentially dangerous and can give rise to a paraplegia. Interruption of all the nerve roots can occur by backward projection of the nucleus pulposus into the spinal canal. Such patients may suffer urinary or faecal retention and loss of sexual function. It is always vital therefore to ask about bladder and bowel function and to test for anal tone and perineal sensation.

Most intervertebral disc prolapses will settle spontaneously after rest, but the effect of the loss of nucleus pulposus and the continued pressure from body weight above will cause a reduction in the height of the disc. This compresses the intervertebral space and the facet joints posteriorly and alters the biomechanics of the vertebral column, giving rise to chronic back pain. The characteristic feature radiographically is of osteophytes at the margins of the vertebral bodies.

Facet joint pain

This is one of the clearest syndromes of back pain and is typically an acute exacerbation of an underlying spondylotic spine. Pain is experienced on extension of the spine,

Table 24.1 Consequences of disc prolapse at various levels

Disc prolapse	Affected nerve root	Loss of reflex	Dermatome	Typical muscle weakness
L3/4	L4	Knee jerk	L4—play a part of anterior aspect of knee and medial aspect of lower leg down to ankle.	Quadriceps muscle, partial tibialis anterior, tibialis posterior
L4/5	L5		Postero-lateral aspect of thigh, lateral aspect of lower leg, dorsum and medial aspect of foot including the medial 3½ toes	Foot dorsiflexors and evertors. Tibialis posterior
L5/S1	S1	Ankle jerk	Small strip of posterior aspect of thigh and posterior aspect of calf, heel and lateral aspect of foot including lateral 1½ toes	Foot plantar flexors, lateral hamstrings and thigh abductors (gluteus maximus)

both in an upright position and in sitting, and can be provoked on bending forwards. The pain often radiates to the buttock or into the sacrum and may extend down the leg but rarely extends beyond the knee. This is not nerve root pain. Flexion of the spine causes pain in distinction from that of intervertebral disc prolapse.

Spondylosis
This is the end result of degenerative changes in the spine and may occur in the facet joints, in the vertebral bodies, and wherever movement of the spine takes place. There is dysfunction of all the structures, which causes chronic low-grade pain. Acute exacerbations occur and treatment is with analgesia and gentle mobilization of the spine. If stiffness occurs, hydrotherapy can be of great use. Patients with chronic pain may benefit from anti-depressant medication and physical measures, such as transcutaneous nerve stimulation, which are dealt with in more detail in Chapter 11.

Spondylolisthesis and spondylolysis
This describes a displacement of one vertebra on another. This is usually anterior movement of a vertebra above on the one below, but posterior movement of the vertebra above on that below can also occur and is referred to as retrolisthesis. Spondylolysis occurs when the spondylolisthesis is caused by a defect in the pars inter-articularis in the vertebral lamina. The treatment for this is usually conservative. Fixation of the spine at that level using a corset or plaster jacket may improve symptoms, if they are very bad and if nerve root compression takes place. In this situation, spinal fusion may be considered as a definitive procedure. The symptoms are very similar to that of facet joint pain.

Spinal stenosis
Chronic disease of the spine can cause narrowing of the spinal canal. This may be due to recurrent disc prolapse and loss of disc height or by facet joint arthritis impinging into the spinal canal. Similarly, the spinal foramen may be narrowed and embarrassed. Symptoms usually start in later life and back and leg pain occur with physical activity. The

condition of spinal claudication typifies the onset of nerve root pain in the leg occurring during physical activity. The symptoms then settle at rest in most patients. It is also found that flexion of the spine relieves the symptoms and walking up hills and going up stairs is often more comfortable than on the flat or going downhill. MR scanning confirms the level of narrowing and, if the patient's symptoms are severe enough and he or she is fit, then a laminectomy is the treatment of choice for full resolution of symptoms.

Management

Acute exacerbation of chronic back pain

Most acute back pain will resolve spontaneously after a few days or weeks and patients should be helped with analgesics. It is essential to rule out underlying inflammatory or neoplastic causes, and if the history and clinical findings do not do this, then further investigation is required through assay of inflammatory markers in the blood. Imaging in simple acute back pain is of little help, but may give an indication of previous underlying disease, such as lumbar spondylosis or osteoporosis.

Leg pain and sciatica may be helped by an epidural injection through either a lumbar or caudal route. Similarly, an acute exacerbation of facet joint pain, in which there is a local tenderness of one and no more than two joints, will be greatly eased by local infiltration of corticosteroid and local anaesthetic. Exercises such as Maitland's and McKenzie mobilizations have been shown to be useful, but no more effective than other forms of treatment. The aim is to relieve the pressure on the spinal structures and rest and cessation of the incriminating factors will usually settle the situation. The use of isokinetic devices to help restore mechanical function appears to be useful, but needs further study. Figure 24.2 gives a management algorithm for an acute back pain service.

Chronic back pain

The management of chronic back pain relies on patient education and the development of a realistic approach to

What is back pain due to?

A problem in the back

A problem elsewhere (e.g. GU, systemic) —— Yes —→ Diagnose and manage appropriately

Is there a spinal cord or cauda equina lesion? —— Yes —→ Emergency referral to spinal surgeon

Sphincter disturbance
Gait disturbance
Saddle anaesthesia

No

Back pain diagnostic triage

Possible serious spinal pathology

Red Flags
Onset age<20 or>55
Non-mechanical pain
PH carcinoma, steroids, HIV
Thoracic pain
Unwell, weight loss
Widespread neurology
Structural deformity

Nerve root problem

Unilateral leg pain
Radiates to foot or toes
Numbness and anaesthesia in
same distribution
SLR reproduces leg pain
Localized neurology

Simple back pain

Onset age 20–55
Lumbosacral, buttocks and thighs
Mechanical pain
Patient well

Is there severe or progressive motor weakness?

Yes

No —→ Primary care management

Urgent specialist referral

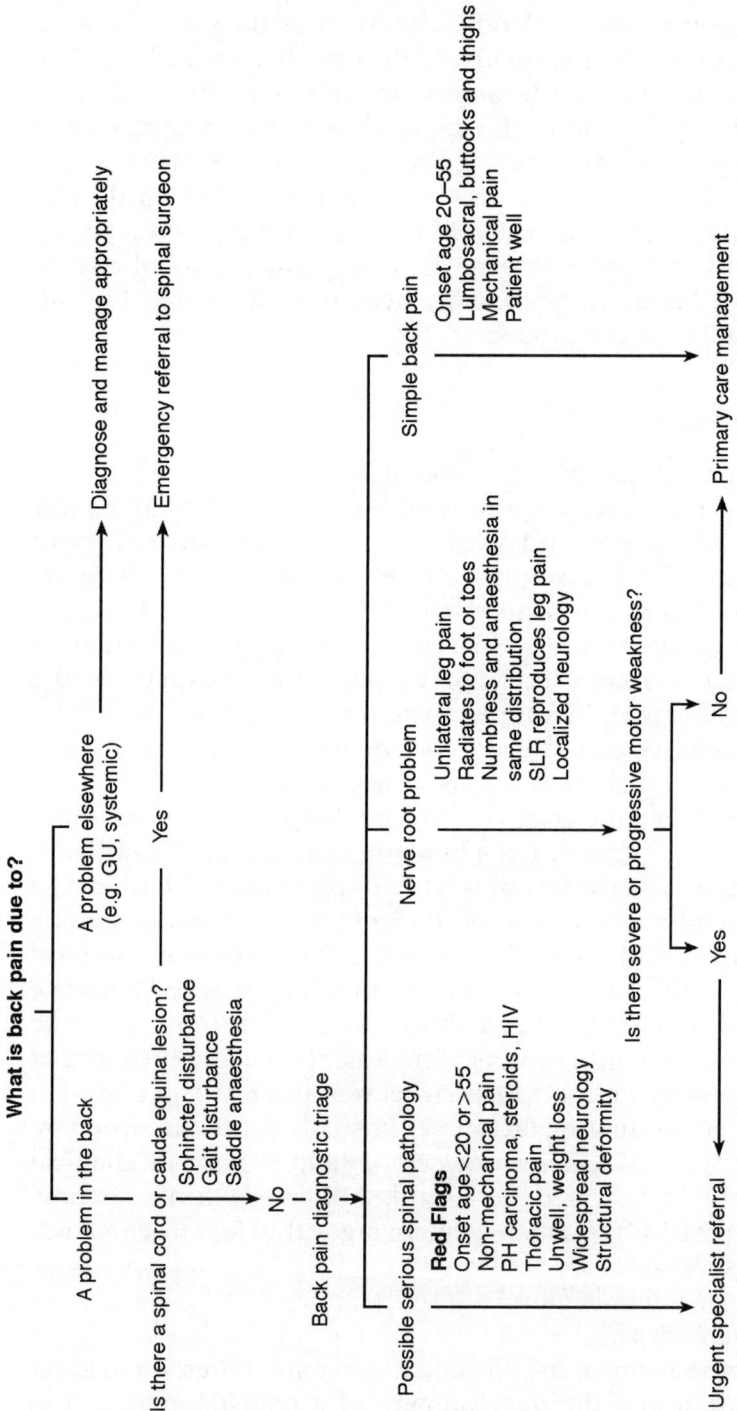

Fig. 24.2(a)   GP diagnostic triage.

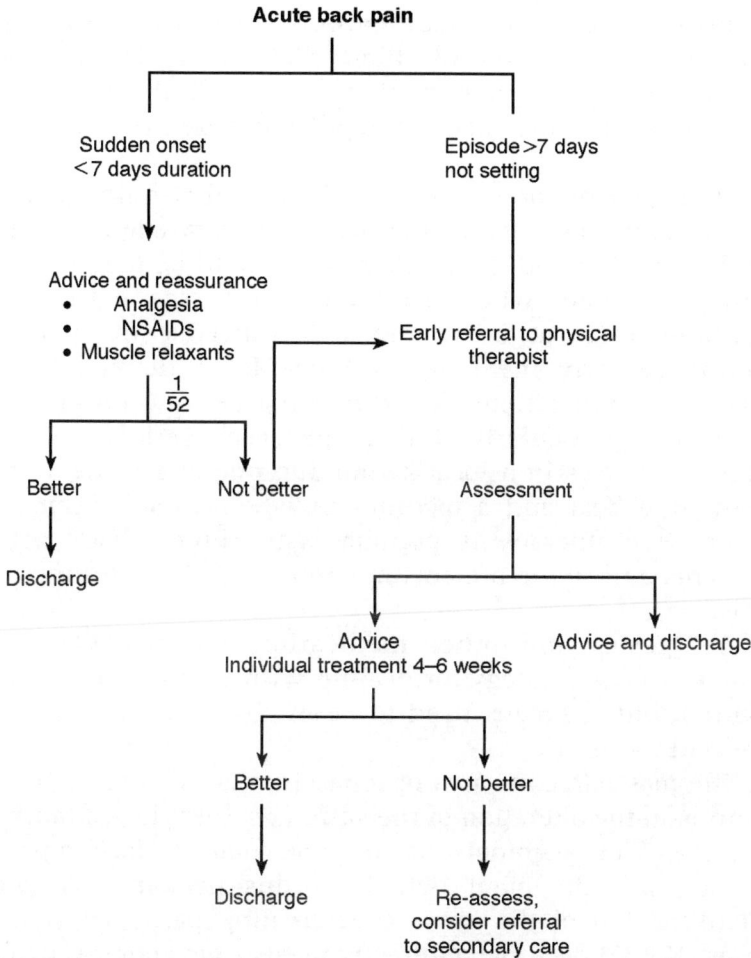

Fig. 24.2(b)   Back pain service—primary care management.

lifestyle management. It is important to separate the
management of acute exacerbations of pain from the chronic
background discomfort which patients suffer. While the
help of doctors and therapists is useful for the former, they
can have a negative impact on the latter. Once it is clear that
a patient has chronic back pain of a mechanical nature, then
a suitable regimen of analgesics and therapies is required.
Thereafter, the role of health professionals should diminish
and patients should not be reliant on continued medical

follow-up. They should be encouraged to be directed to further rehabilitation for their social and occupational needs and further investigations and medical treatments/ therapies will only increase dependence on the find for a 'cure'.

Management should therefore be aimed at mild, gentle, but effective exercise to improve muscle strength and to mobilize the spine. These exercises should be taught by a physiotherapist, who will then require the patient to continue them at home and will supervise the latter's ability to carry them out at home for a defined time. Thereafter, the patient should be expected to continue the exercises, particularly during quiescent periods. Warm water exercises in a local swimming pool are valuable in providing heat and a medium in which exercise can be done. Hydrotherapy is popular with chronic back pain patients and spa treatments in continental Europe support this.

Analgesics and other medication are discussed in Chapter 11. A strategy for dealing with chronic pain is required, but regimens need to be established for patient's individual needs.

The most effective area of rehabilitation in chronic back pain is in the alteration of the sufferer's lifestyle. Certainly, the use of a psychologist has become commonplace in pain clinics, but the main benefit of this person is in the identification of the key issues creating particular problems. Not all back pain sufferers needs psychological help, but do need a strategy in which to cope with their symptoms. They need clear instructions about their daily routines and dealing with acute exacerbations. This can be done by a clinical psychologist, but other team members are also able to give such advice. One of the real values of a clinical psychologist is in the organization of multi-disciplinary team work, so that consistent messages are given to patients and relatives. Therapy is essentially reserved for acute exacerbations under clear and reasonably strict criteria. The team should also involve the primary care team, social services and the Disability Employment Adviser. Alterations to the home, workplace, and transportation are important and back pain sufferers should be encouraged to take up activities which will not cause particularly difficulties for their symptoms.

Our experience is that back pain classes are useful for people at risk. Their value is unproven for established back pain sufferers, but may allow a better appreciation of prevention of exacerbations through peer support.

Occupational advice has been variable over the years and placement and counselling teams (PACTS) can provide help for companies as well as individual back pain sufferers through Disability Employment Advisers.

Conclusion

Back pain is an enormous problem for which there are few straightforward answers. However, a systemic approach to sufferers can be adopted by health professionals and clear communication between these players is vital for optimal management.

Neck pain

Neck pain is another common musculoskeletal problem presenting to GPs, therapists, rheumatologists, and orthopaedic surgeons as well as rehabilitation physicians. The principle of managing chronic neck pain is similar to that of managing chronic back pain and strategies are discussed in more detail in Chapter 11. However, the management of acute neck pain is important in this context, particularly where acute on chronic symptoms exist.

Clinical features

Neck problems usually present with pain and stiffness and are often associated with some unaccustomed activity, awkward posture, or injury, but specific insult is not necessarily required. Pain is often felt in the back of the lower part of the neck and can radiate up to the occiput, down the spine or to the shoulders, and down the arms. As in lumbar spine disease, nerve root compression can occur and this is most commonly seen in the C7 dermatome.

Symptoms are usually aggravated by movement of the neck and relieved by rest. Most acute exacerbations of neck pain last for no more than a few days. Where a specific injury has been involved, the duration of symptoms obviously depends on the severity, but, in the absence of disruption of the ligamentous structures to the spine, should settle within a few weeks. Following a whiplash injury in road traffic accidents, one appreciates that there may be anterior neck pain for several months and the absence of nerve root involvement, a full range of neck movements on active and passive examination would suggest complete resolution of the neck pain symptoms. Certainly, from a medico-legal point of view, one would not expect the symptoms in these patients to persist for more than two years and would not give rise to subsequent degenerative change. Symptoms and signs are given in Table 24.2 and the associated features of nerve root involvement are also given in Table 24.3.

The main differentiation between neck pain of mechanical origin and of inflammatory origin (e.g. in rheumatoid disease, ankylosing spondylitis) is that the former produces asymmetric restriction of movement, whereas the latter tends to be symmetrical. Because of the large number of

Table 24.2 Symptoms and signs

Problem	Symptoms	Signs
Articular	Intermittent neck pain	Asymmetrical restriction of neck movement
Dural	Pain in occiput, vertex, scapula, shoulder, and interscapula	Pain may occur on shoulder adduction or external rotation, but pain on forced lateral flexion of cervical spine
Nerve root	Severe pain in appropriate dermatome	Weakness and sensory impairment in affected nerve root distribution, abnormal reflex if necessary

Table 24.3 Cervical root signs and symptoms

Root	Pain distribution	Muscle weakness	Tendon reflex
C2	Occiput radiating over head to forehead		
C3	Neck, jaw, and cheek		
C4	Trapezius and upper medial border of scapula		
C5	Shoulder tip, lateral side of upper arm	Supraspinatus, infraspinatus, deltoid, biceps	Biceps
C6	Front of arm, lateral aspect of elbow, and radial border of forearm down to thumb	Biceps supinator	Supinator
C7	Middle of anterior and posterior aspects of forearm, middle and ring fingers	Triceps, wrist flexors	Triceps
C8	Ulnar aspect of forearm and hand, ring and little finger	Wrist and finger flexors, thumb flexors	
T1	Medial aspect of elbow. Upper pectoral and mid scapula areas	Intrinsic hand muscles	
T2	Medial aspect of upper arm and axilla		

causes of neck pain, it is important to identify those in which concern should be raised. Table 24.4 shows some of these features.

Treatment

Most neck pain is usually self-limiting, treatment is usually supportive and relies on analgesics. Rest, perhaps with use of a soft collar, can be helpful, but care is needed in the fitting of these devices, so that the spine is supported in a neutral position. The aim is to restrict neck movements to about one-third, and, while rigid collars can achieve reduction to about 10 per cent, they are cumbersome and uncomfortable to wear. They should thus be reserved for patients at risk of neurological compression. Physiotherapy and chiropracty are commonly performed and traction can be used when root pain occurs. This can be carried out in a lying or sitting position with sufficient force to overcome gravity and muscle and joint resistance. Mobilization exercises and manipulation are also performed where cervical joints are repeatedly pressed through their ranges of movement. Manipulation is simply a more energetic and aggressive form of mobilization and older patients should not generally be subjected to it.

Table 24.4   Symptoms and signs in neck pain

Class of symptom	Details
Symptoms suggestive of a mechanical cause	Intermittent symptoms Pain confined to articular and dural distribution Neurological features confined to a single root
Worrying symptoms	Constant or progressive symptoms Neurological features, bilateral or involving more than one nerve root

X-rays show typical features of cervical spondylosis with osteophyte formation, as in Figs. 24.3(a) and 24.3(b).

Because neck pain can become chronic and very disabling, many other associated features can develop, which are discussed in more detail in Chapter 11.

Shoulder pain

Soft tissue rheumatism presenting as shoulder pain is a common presentation and may or may not occur after trauma. Referred pain from the neck should be considered before attending to the shoulder structures themselves. The upper limb is suspended from the trunk by muscular attachments and thus any condition affecting muscular strength or function may cause pain. In this respect, the shoulder is completely different from lower limb joints, and is not designed in humans to bear weight. Therefore, neuromuscular loss, for instance from an impaired C5 cervical root, will lead to marked loss of function and it is important to know not only the anatomy of the brachial plexus, but the spinal root innervation of muscles in the upper limb. This is one of the keys to success in treating painful upper limb syndromes.

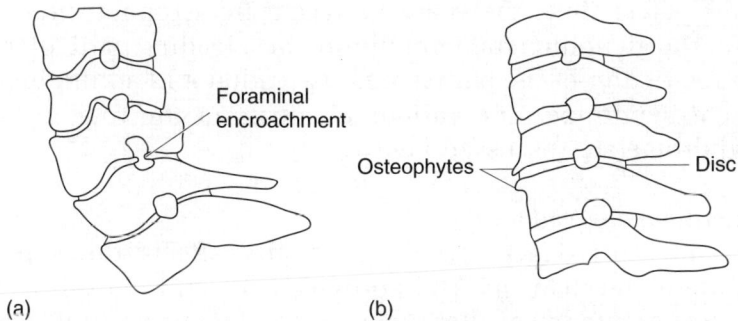

Foraminal encroachment

Osteophytes — Disc

(a)   (b)

Fig. 24.3 (a) Showing oblique views of cervical spine, highlighting foraminal encroachment by osteophytes; (b) Showing loss of cervical lordosis, reduction in disc space, and anterior and posterior osteophyte formation.

Shoulder pain classically occurs on movement or when lying on the affected side at night. Another common feature is a painful arc syndrome, which causes discomfort as the shoulder is raised in abduction and, as the movement continues, the pain then disappears. Examination of the shoulder can give rise to some confusing problems, particularly in the domain of tenderness. Deep palpation of a normal shoulder will usually be tender. The coracoid process is often tender, for instance in supraspinatus tendinitis, which may be confused with a bicipital tendinitis.

A shoulder must keep moving to maintain function and a fall may produce supraspinatus tendon impingement and extreme pain, such that the patient stops moving the limb. The restriction of movement can lead very quickly on to a true frozen shoulder, i.e. an adhesive capsulitis. Three distinct syndromes exist in the painful shoulder, which are as follows.

Rotator cuff lesions

Movement of the arm around the shoulder occurs as a result of a group of muscles working together (Table 24.5). They can suffer injury as a result of falls onto an outstretched hand, or suffer minor recurrent damage producing degenerative change. A rotator cuff syndrome may occur as a result of vascular changes and mechanical factors affecting normal muscular and tendon function which produces pain. Over time, the space between the acromion process and the glenohumeral joint diminishes, leading particularly to restriction of the supraspinatus tendon and an impingement syndrome. The various elements of the rotator cuff syndrome are discussed below.

Supraspinatus tendinitis
Rotator cuff degeneration principally affects the supraspinatus mechanism. The portion of the cuff closest to its insertion into the greater tuberosity and pain and limitation of active and passive abduction is characteristic. A painful arc occurs on abduction between 90° and 120°. The pain may be increased on resisting abduction of the arm in the first 15° of movement by placing the examiner's hand on

Table 24.5 Rotator cuff muscles

Muscle	Action	Innervation
Deltoid	Abduction and flexion of arm 15–90°	Axillary Nerve
Supraspinatus	Abduction of arm 0–15° and 90° upwards	Suprascapular nerve
Infraspinatus	External rotation of arm	Suprascapular nerve
Subscapularis	Internal rotation of arm	Suprascapular nerve
Serratus anterior	Protraction of arm	Long thoracic nerve
Biceps brachii, long head	Forearm supination and elbow and shoulder flexion	Musculocutaneous nerve
Pectoralis major	Adduction of arm	Long thoracic nerve
Teres major & minor	Adduction of arm	Axillary nerve
Latissimus dorsi	Extension of shoulders	Thoracodorsal nerve
Rhomboids	Extension of shoulders	Dorsal scapular nerve

the elbow and asking the patient to abduct the arm against the examiner's hand on the elbow.

Calcific tendinitis
Some cases of supraspinatus tendinitis occur acutely and are associated with calcium deposits which are seen on x-ray. These are often associated with a very severe rotator cuff pain when the deposits are extravasated into the sub-acromial bursa and can lead to chronic inflammation of the tendon. Treatment by injection into the subacromial bursa is often effective.

Infraspinatus and subscapularis tendinitis
Although less common than supraspinatus tendinitis, these two lesions give distinctive features. Both cause pain on abduction of the arm, but the former gives rise to pain on external rotation of the arm and the latter to pain on internal rotation of the arm. The former is more common in sportsmen than other lesions of the rotator cuff.

Bicipital tendinitis
This produces pain anteriorly on the shoulder in the area where the bicipital tendon passes through the groove in the humeral head to a detachment in the coracoid process. Chronic tendinitis can give rise to rupture of the tendon. Local injection may be helpful.

Subacromial bursitis
This somewhat non-specific term describes a rotator cuff problem, where the specific tendon lesion is not readily identifiable. The pain is most commonly evident on abduction and on flexion of the arm and both may be restricted, but stressing the individual tendons may not produce intense pain in one area more than others. The most common feature is of a painful arc around 45° to 60° of abduction.

Adhesive capsulitis—frozen shoulder

This occurs either spontaneously or following rotator cuff lesions and is more common in diabetics and following immobility from causes other than trauma. Patients following stroke may certainly develop an intense adhesive capsulitis, which can arise from injudicious nursing of patients or from spasticity causing decreased movement in the shoulder. It is most important for nurses to ensure that the shoulder is not damaged during the early phase of stroke care when the limb is flaccid, because moving patients around beds and chairs by placing an arm under the axilla can tear the capsule. Additionally, patients following myocardial infarction, pericarditis, and thoracotomy (particularly sternal splits) can suffer an intense adhesive capsulitis, which responds very well to physical treatment and to injection.

The essential features of adhesive capsulitis are an inflamed capsule of the gleno-humeral joint which eventually shrinks and thickens, thus restricting movement. Abduction is restricted in common with rotator cuff lesions, but the pathognomonic feature and main difference is that external rotation is preferentially restricted compared to rotator cuff lesions. Early treatment is important, as a secondary reflex sympathetic dystrophy can occur, leading to a useless arm and hand, which will be very difficult to treat.

Acromioclavicular joint lesions

Men and women in their 40s and 50s may develop degenerative changes in the acromioclavicular joint. Sportsmen and manual workers are particularly affected and injury can give rise to subluxation or even dislocation. It is characterized by tenderness over the joint and by pain on stressing flexion and abduction of the arm between 60° and 90°. Radiographs show typical degenerative changes with loss of joint space and possibly osteophyte formation. Inferiorly placed osteophytes can in themselves impinge the rotator cuff by encroaching into the subacromial space.

Treatment of shoulder pain

Treatment of these lesions is essentially with analgesics and physiotherapy to mobilize the joint. NSAIDs are of little use and it may be necessary to use quite strong analgesics to allow sleep. Rotator cuff lesions may respond to an injection of steroid and local anaesthetic into the subacromial bursa and adhesive capsulitis responds by the similar infiltration into the glenohumeral joint itself. If rotator cuff lesions persist and are clearly due to impingement, it may be necessary after MR scanning (which gives brilliant images of the shoulder) to decompress the space surgically. Injection of the acromioclavicular joint can be very effective if the pain emanates from there. Similarly, the distal end of the clavicle may require removal in persistent severe acromioclavicular joint pain.

The principle of treating adhesive capsulitis is to mobilize the joint as much as possible by physical means and to utilize injections to allow physical treatment to be taken further. If this is not possible, manipulation of the joint under anaesthetic has no proven effect, but is useful in some patients, as long as an intensive series of physiotherapy treatments is planned for five days immediately after the procedure. The prognosis is in fact very good for all these lesions.

Epicondylitis at the elbow

Tennis elbow (lateral humeral epicondylitis) and golfer's elbow (medial humeral epicondylitis) are two annoying conditions and are thought to be part of an overuse syndrome. Both result from excessive tension on the common forearm extensor and flexor muscles respectively and result in localized tenderness and pain. They often prevent function of the hand, particularly in lifting weights and may be associated with neck pain, which needs to be treated beforehand. Both usually present in people over the age of 40 and may co-exist. The pain may be severe enough to prevent sleep and is usually aggravated by gripping and twisting. It is common in manual occupations where gripping and twisting are necessary and the syndrome only rarely occurs in either tennis or golf.

To elucidate the clinical signs, the patient should be seated and the elbow is palpated over the lateral or humeral epicondyles for tenderness. In tennis elbow, intense pain is brought on by resisted extension of the wrist and fingers with the arm supported with a straight elbow. Similarly, forced pronation of the forearm with the elbow straight also produces pain. In contrast, a straight arm and resisted wrist flexion and finger flexion produces pain over the medial humeral epicondyle in golfer's elbow. The association with painful supination is less reliable and sensory symptoms do not typically occur. The diagnosis is clinical and imaging only serves to rule out underlying degenerative disease at the radio-humeral joint.

Atypical features are seen in these conditions as listed below, and are usually suggestive of a manifestation of problems from elsewhere:

1. Bilateral symptoms and signs, or the presence of both golfer's and tennis elbow.
2. No epicondylar tenderness.
3. Paraesthesiae in the arm and painful limitation of neck movements, associated with nerve root disturbance.
4. Failure to respond to local injection or occurrence within a week or two of injection.
5. Clinical or radiological evidence of arthritis at the elbow.

Treatment

Physical treatment is usually helpful in cases of mild epicondylitis. No one particular treatment has been shown to be superior to another. Use of an epicondylitis clasp can protect the common muscular origin by a subtle change of forces on the musculo-tendinous junction. A clasp is worn reasonably tightly around the upper forearm just below the common extensor or common flexor origin and the forces are transmitted away from the bony-ligamentous attachment. This can usefully allow people to continue to work. If these measures are not sufficient, local injection of hydrocortisone is very useful in diminishing and treating symptoms. Hydrocortisone alone should be used in preference to fluorinated corticosteroids, as the latter may cause subcutaneous fat atrophy and local disfigurement.

Carpal tunnel syndrome

This condition is due to entrapment of the median nerve as

it passes through the carpal tunnel under the flexor retinaculum at the wrist. It is usually idiopathic and may be associated with expansion of the long flexor tendons, but may occur secondarily to other conditions. The commonest cause is due to fluid retention in women who are either pregnant or on the oral contraceptive; some of the causes are listed below:

- Fluid retention—pregnancy or oral contraceptive
- Osteoarthritis or rheumatoid arthritis of the wrist
- Fractures around the wrist—colles and scaphoid fractures
- Direct trauma
- Hypothyroidism
- Acromegaly
- Amyloidosis
- Scheie's syndrome
- Myelomatosis.

Clinical features

Pain and paraesthesiae occurring in the territory of the median nerve are the classic features, i.e. in the radial aspect of the palmar surface of the hand to include the lateral 3½ fingers. Pain typically comes on at night when sleeping posture often results in either flexion or extension of the wrist, thereby increasing the pressure within the carpal tunnel. Patients often wake up and gain relief by hanging their hand out of bed, which cools the limb and therefore reduces the symptoms. In more severe cases, motor involvement occurs with weakness and atrophy of abductor pollicis brevis. The diagnosis is made by examination and confirmed by a positive Tinel's sign where percussion of the nerve at the wrist produces pain and paraesthesiae in the median nerve territory. A similar result may also be achieved by sustained full flexion or extension of the wrist (Phalen's sign). Nerve conduction studies and electromyography of the abductor pollicis brevis muscle give the diagnosis and differentiates it from compression of the median nerve elsewhere.

Treatment is by resting the wrist in a volar splint in mild cases to prevent excessive extension and flexion. This is often sufficient, but local injection of hydrocortisone, particularly in arthritis, will often achieve good results. Where symptoms are severe and where active denervation is present, decompression of the carpal tunnel can be effected by removal of a strip of the flexor retinaculum. The prognosis is excellent and recovery is swift.

De Quervain's stenosing tenosynovitis

This is due to inflammation of abductor pollicis longus and extensor pollicis brevis tendon sheaths in the wrist and the characteristic pain on the radial aspect of the wrist is often a feature of occupational activity. There is local tenderness and a positive Finkelstein's test will give a clue to the diagnosis. This is carried out by flexion and opposition of the thumb into the palm of the hand and held down by the fingers. The wrist is then subjected to an ulnar deviation force, thus stretching the affected tendons and producing pain. Treatment is again through local injection of hydrocortisone, although physical measures can be successful. Protection of the wrist in a Futuro wrist splint is very helpful, particularly where occupational activities have been incriminated.

Work related upper limb disorders

This is a wide and controversial area of clinical practice and is often associated with personal injury litigation. This will not be discussed in detail, but a full account is available in the suggested further reading.

Further reading

ARC booklets on back pain. Arthritis and Rheumatism Council, 41 Eagle Street, London.

Barnes, M. P., Braithwaite, B., and Ward, A. B. (1997). *The medical aspects of personal injury litigation*. Blackwell Scientific, Oxford.

Clinical Standards Advisory Group Guidelines on Back Pain. London. HMSO. 1994.

....

Disc disorders. a handbook for patients. Arthritis and Rheumatism
　　Council, 41 Eagle Street, London.
Manual handling regulations, 1992. HMSO, London.

Useful address

National Back Pain Association
16 Elm Tree Road
Teddington
Middlesex TW11 8ST, UK

25

....

Amputation

The rehabilitation of amputees is a major activity within rehabilitation medicine. Amputee care covers a range of conditions from congenital limb deficiency to the effects of peripheral vascular disease and diabetes in older patients. This chapter will provide the reader with some basic principles of the care of the amputee and of prosthetic fitting for deficient limbs from no matter what cause.

Epidemiology

The major cause of amputation in the UK is arteriosclerotic peripheral vascular disease followed by diabetes. Hypertension, obesity, diabetes itself, hyperlipidaemia, and, above all, smoking, are the main elements behind the development of peripheral vascular disease and, despite improved techniques in arterial bypass operations, amputation is still routinely performed in the developed world. It is an operation of middle or later years and the common pathological processes are end-stage obliterative arterial disease and the micro-angiopathic and neurological consequences of diabetes. Trauma and infection are still major causes in the developing world. Table 25.1 shows the aetiology behind amputation by age group.

Table 25.1 Amputations by age and cause

Aetiology	Age (years)					
	0–9	10–19	29–39	40–59	60–79	80+
Trauma	1	33	158	93	41	7
Vascular	2	0	17	294	1563	323
Diabetic	2	0	5	140	507	68
Infection	1	0	13	13	28	2
Malignancy	0	11	26	28	37	10

About 5000 patients are referred annually in the UK for prosthetic treatment following about 10 000 amputations and certainly the impression nowadays is that patients are referred for amputation later, as some have previously had arterial surgery.

In comparison to lower limb amputation and amputee rehabilitation, upper limb amputation is quite uncommon and forms only about 10 per cent of the total activity. Amputations from trauma and congenital limb deficiency are in themselves uncommon in the UK, but, as they occur in younger people, they are likely to have a relatively greater impact on the service, as the users will need an artificial limb for longer, and may have more demanding expectations to allow them to return to an active life. Regular limb changes will be required in growing children and, during growth spurts, they may need to be seen every three or four months.

Planning an amputation

The great majority of amputations are carried out as elective procedures and can therefore be planned, not only surgically, but from the rehabilitation view as well. This process should begin as soon as amputation is considered and is involved with the education of the patient, the realization of realistic expectations and, if the patient is to be able to use an artificial limb, the fitting of a limb and the physical rehabilitation before and after. Amputee care teams are now set up between groups of professionals, involving the vascular surgeon, the physician in rehabilitation medicine, nurses, physiotherapists, occupational therapists, prosthetists, and clinical psychologists. Good liaison should be developed with the local wheelchair service and the whole process should centre on the rehabilitation activity. Patients will have many needs in respect of their disability, of which one will be for an artificial limb. The rehabilitation team should advise the surgeon on the practicalities of individual patients being able to tolerate artificial limbs and the choice of surgical operation should match these requirements.

Following the operation, the general practitioner and social services should be involved in the transfer of care from the surgical team to that of the rehabilitation physician, specialist physiotherapist, prosthetist, and chiropodist, who will continue the rehabilitation process. All major lower limb amputees will need a wheelchair early on following operation and a significant proportion of elderly amputees will use wheelchair mobility at least for some of the day.

The amputee should be introduced to the amputee care team in the limb fitting centre, for he or she will require their help and support for the rest of his/her life. Even once independence has been achieved, repeated visits will be required for maintenance and adjustment of the prosthesis.

Information is the key to success, as in so many aspects of rehabilitation, and this should start in the pre-amputation consultations with the vascular surgeon and the rehabilitation team. Description of what it is like to be an amputee and of phantom limb pain and phantom sensation are vital to allow those patients to cope with these very real difficulties. Most amputees will suffer some phantom pain and phantom limb sensation to a greater or lesser degree and falls are not infrequent in the first few weeks following the procedure, when an attempt is made to stand for transfers or for walking. This can damage the stump and awareness of the absent limb needs to be made. Phantom limb pain is associated with pain pre-operatively, and sustained pain relief for at least 72 hours before the operation, reduces it symptomatology. Epidural injections may be of value in achieving this. Certainly, if epidural anaesthesia is to be used, it should be started 24 hours before surgery and maintained for about 48 hours afterwards.

Amputation care

In order to allow somebody to walk effectively following amputation, the patient must be generally fit and well. In view of the fact that most patients are elderly and have had peripheral vascular disease or diabetes for many years, their fitness is often below par. Therefore, fitness training is required to allow them to have sufficient strength to transfer and to stand for long periods. Most importantly, care of the surviving limb is vital, as it too can become damaged from the underlying disease process, and it must be sufficiently resilient to withstand increased activity. For this reason, hopping and jumping should be avoided in order not to damage the foot.

The level of surgery is critical for the expected level of independence that may ultimately be achieved. The surgeon naturally has to carry out an operation which will immediately ensure good circulation and healing in the stump as well as provide a base upon which the patient may then walk again. The most common operations are transtibial and transfemoral amputations in the lower limb and transradial and transhumeral amputations in the upper limb. Amputation through the knee is described as knee disarticulation and all these terms have been subjected to internationally recognized descriptors. Congenital limb deficiency is described under separate descriptors, which date back to 1989. The key element in predicting outcome is the preservation of a functioning knee joint. This reduces the energy cost of walking and allows considerable ease in transfers and in the preservation of cosmesis. Energy consumption is increased in below-knee amputees due to vascular disease by 55 per cent and by 120 per cent in above-knee cases. Bilateral above-knee amputees require 280 per cent more energy for the same activity as an able-bodied person of the same age.

The length of the stump has an effect on the application of the prosthesis. As a general rule, amputation between the

middle and distal thirds of the thigh is ideal for transfemoral amputation and between the proximal and middle
thirds of the tibia for the transtibial level. While disarticulation at the knee is straightforward in operative terms and
provides great potential for force transmission very quickly
after surgery, it causes great difficulty for wearing a prosthesis. Creating an effective joint is difficult and surgeons
have over the years been dissuaded from carrying out this
operation. Where it is clear that the patient will not use an
artificial limb, knee disarticulation or Gritti–Stokes amputation is of greater value, as it confers some benefits to
sitting in an appropriate wheelchair. The stump needs
protection by good quality skin flaps and muscle reattach-
ment should be carried out so that excessive muscular bulk
does not interfere with the socket fitting process. Similarly,
problems arising from poor trimming of bone and nerve
transection are preventable.

The limb fitting process

After surgery, fitting can be expected within 10 to 14 days.
Surgery should take place in designated centres to ensure
good expertise and to ensure integration with the rehabilitation team. The stump should be inspected regularly for
oedema and infection and, at an appropriate time, an early
walking aid will be introduced. The post-amputation
mobility aid (PPAM) is the best known and is often fitted
as early as three to four weeks. It is clearly useful in
allowing compression of the stump through its air cells,
thereby reducing oedema and in promoting healing.
Because it also allows early standing, it is particularly
useful in the elderly, as balance may be lost.

Planning rehabilitation goals is an important and continuous process. As in other forms of rehabilitation, the
views of the patient and carer contribute essentially to the
overall rehabilitation goal and the assessment must look
to all the needs, of which only one will be for mobility.
Therefore medical, nursing, and therapist provision will be
incorporated into the programme along with counselling,
financial, and housing issues.

....

Prosthetic treatment

Stump casting and measurement and limb prescription should
be possible from the 21st post-operative day. Nowadays,
modular systems are used from the very first prescription
and temporary cosmetic covers shorten delivery times. Gait
re-education with the first prosthesis follows a sequence
which is common to all lower limb amputees:
1. Full weight-bearing and weight transfer.
2. Walking within parallel bars, turning by stepping.
3. Walking with sticks between two parallel bars.
4. Walking with one stick between parallel bars.
5. Walking with aids out of the bars.
6. Optimal gait with minimal walking aids.

The prescription of a prosthesis has certain features in
common, which interface with the residual limb:
• Socket structure
• Skeletal structure
• Articular structures
• Terminal structures
• A cosmetic covering
• A suspension

Modern prostheses incorporate considerable design features
to improve the gait cycle and the use of intelligent knees
and ankle shock absorption allow a smoother gait, thereby
reducing the energy cost and improving the quality of gait.
Lower limb prostheses must be able to resist the forces
transmitted during stance and gait without serious risk of
mechanical failure. Functional limb prostheses may be
body powered, although electrically powered features are
now becoming more commonly available.

Great care must be taken of the skin of the stump, which
is in contact with the inner surface of the socket. A variety
of silicones are used in suction and adhesion devices at the
interface, but stump sheaths, called stump socks, are the
commonest interface, as they provide considerable relief
from shear forces. Upper limb prostheses may be cosmetic
or functional and functional types may be fabricated to a
variety of specifications. A battery-powered electric hand
can be controlled by selective contraction of flexor and

extensor muscle groups in the residual limb, but these active devices are expensive and at present do not confer great advantage to the user. However, they are improving all the time.

It is not within the remit of this book to go into great detail on the availability and features of artificial limbs, but suffice it to say that real technical progress has been made with different forms of ankle articulation (e.g. the summit ankle, cushion heel or SACH foot, poly-axial ankles and carbon fibre-based foot/ankle/shin unitary systems). Knee joints may be unicentric or polycentric. A new intelligent knee has now been developed and fitting to modern modular systems has made the limb fitting process relatively straightforward.

One important point to note for non-specialist professionals is that any prosthesis has to allow sufficient height for the foot to swing through during the swing phase of the gait cycle. Therefore, heel strike at the start of the next stance phase has to be controlled very quickly, if the artificial leg is to cope with walking forces and the patient has to have the ability to achieve the correct posture and position.

Special needs

The needs of young people with limb deficiency and the increased interest among disabled people in sporting activities mean that heavy-duty artificial limbs require to be combined with readily adjustable but strong components. Hydraulic swing-phase controls and energy storing and reducing shin/ankle/foot systems are such examples. Both exo- and endoskeletal prostheses are not usually waterproof and so getting wet can prove somewhat hazardous. Protective sleeves are therefore used over the prosthesis for protection.

Outcomes

As in many aspects of disability, it is difficult to find a useful, easily applicable measure of progress during rehabilitation. The Harold Wood/Stanmore Scale and the Guy Scales measure mobility and are currently used in the UK. A Grise Scale is validated as a general outcome measure for amputees, but unfortunately is insensitive to change and it is this very element on which one wishes to gain most information.

Amputees thus require to be subjected to standard rehabilitation outcome measures, along with mobility, impairment, and disability measures.

Conclusions

Amputee care is a major factor in rehabilitation medicine and requires consultant input. A clear objective for rehabilitation is required in all cases and the fitting of an artificial limb is one aspect in the overall needs of the disabled individual. A common-sense approach to amputee rehabilitation is required and close working with many professionals is vital in ensuring that all elements of the process are coordinated to allow amputees to be fit and well-adjusted to regular use of their artificial limbs.

Further reading

Amputee Medical Rehabilitation Society (AMRS) (1992). *Amputee rehabilitation. Recommended standards and guidelines. A report by a working party of the AMRS.* (Copies from AMRS Secretary c/o Royal College of Physicians, 11 St Andrews Place, Regents Park, London NW1 4LE, UK.)

Bowker, J. H. and Michael, J. W. (ed.) (1992). *Atlas of limb prosthetics.* Mosby Year Books, London.

Bowker, J. H. and Michael, J. W. (1992). *Atlas of limb prosthetics: surgical prosthetics and rehabilitation principles.* Mosby, St Louis.

26

....

Ageing and disability

Two aspects of ageing need to be considered in physically disabled people. The first is the impact of the disability on the ageing process and the second is, vice versa, the impact of the ageing process on disabled people. Because of increasing longevity, the number of people with chronic disease who require care and intermittent rehabilitation increases accordingly, putting great pressure on beds in the National Health Service. The range of disorders and their impact on the individual is similar to that in younger age groups, and produces similar levels of disability in all ages. The considerable variation in the needs of elderly people compared to their younger peers often relates as much to the family support mechanisms as to the understanding of disease process and just because a condition appears in older people, it does not necessarily mean that it will follow a similar course to younger affected patients.

The main element therefore is to identify age changes which occur in the life of the elderly compared with that of younger age groups.

Effects of age on disability

Are there any differences between the ageing process in disabled and able-bodied individuals? The answer is probably no, but there are specific features which seem to occur more readily in disabled people. People now surviving longer with disability seek increased help from health and social services. Their ability to maintain independence does change with increasing age (as does the rest of the population's) and this is often manifest in the need for increased care and an up-grading of equipment levels and complexity accordingly.

The most common aspect of the ageing process in physically disabled people is the appearance of degenerative joint disease. People who may have been managing reasonably well, become decompensated by painful joints. They thus are unable to take as much exercise and to carry out as much activity as before and thus become deconditioned physically and mentally, which then leads to decreased fitness. The more serious effects include an increased prevalence of shoulder, hip, and knee osteoarthritis in comparison to the general population with radiological changes in 54 per cent of men and 58 per cent of women. Joint pain and soreness has also been reported and decreased strength and energy levels are noted, particularly in tetraplegics.

Specific examples of ageing features in disability

There are a few classic examples of the effects of ageing in people with long-standing disabilities. The most obvious example is the increasing number of comorbidities leading to difficulties in concentrating on the rehabilitation process.

Spinal injuries

The effects of ageing in spinal cord injury are now being seen, as patients survive with tetra- and paraplegias. Shoulder and neck problems appear to be evident from years of wheelchair propulsion and from the effect of using the upper limbs as weight-bearing structures. A significant proportion require surgery to correct rotator cuff lesions and there is an increased incidence of pressure sores with increasing age. Cardiopulmonary impairments develop and are evident with impaired circulation in the legs and hypertension in tetraplegics. Paraplegics have a profile consistent with the general population. Mortality increases exponentially with age, but there is an extra mortality due to spinal cord injury. However, the mortality ratio decreases with age. Whereas a 20 year old with a spinal cord injury has a mortality eight times higher than the general population, survivors aged 70 years have a mortality rate of only 1.5 times higher. It was reported that the causes of death mirrored the general population and that there was an association with renal failure, particularly again in tetraplegics. However, over the years, since these studies have become more widely known, renal problems have been better addressed and the mortality is much more akin to the non-disabled population.

Mobility

The normal ageing process changes one's gait throughout life. As one passes from an infant's gait, which is wide-based and involves pelvic rotation, myelination allows better neuromuscular transmission and growth of bones allows an adult-type gait at around the age of the fifth birthday. Serially, as one gets older, balance mechanisms become less efficient and one naturally shortens the stride length in walking and increases the proportion of the stance phase during the gait cycle during the seventh decade of life. This ensures better stability while walking, but results in decreased walking speed and shortened strides. Increased loading of joints leads to degenerative change in the hip and knee. Similarly, the vectors of the forces coming up the lower limb during this altered gait cycle lead to mild flexion of the trunk, which over years, gives the stooped posture of elderly people. This puts increasing pressure on the articulating facet joints in the lumbar spine, and hence the stiffness and discomfort that can develop.

Traumatic brain injury

There are two age-related peaks in the incidence of traumatic brain injury. In the young, injuries occur from car accidents, etc., but in the elderly they are often due to falls within the home. With multisystem failure, the mobility and stability of people decreases and they fall over more readily. This then can result in head injuries and is a reflection more of their social and health status rather than the epidemic seen in younger people. However, as with the young, physical and cognitive changes occur to an already failing brain and there is a significant morbidity and mortality attached to traumatic brain injury in the elderly. Additionally less force is required to damage the skull bones, but elderly people somewhat paradoxically appear to recover better than expected both cognitively and physically after traumatic brain injury.

Post-polio syndrome

This syndrome is classically seen 20 or so years after the development of poliomyelitis-related disability. People with poliomyelitis learn to cope with their disability while young, but after a while, they notice increasing difficulty carrying out tasks which were previously straightforward and further investigation shows denervation in the muscles supplied by the affected anterior horn cells. In simplistic terms, it would appear that their lower motor neurons 'burn out' after years of 'overwork' and this possibly represents the effect of normal ageing on a depleted population of anterior horn cells, which have had to supply an expanded number of motor units. There is no evidence that this syndrome has been caused by an awakening of any viral activity in the disease.

Conclusions

There is an increased incidence of musculoskeletal disease, in strokes, in neurodegenerative disease, and in cancers, with increasing age. As stated earlier, the rehabilitation of older people is complicated by the presence of comorbidities which slow the rehabilitation process down and is one of the major differences between rehabilitating the elderly population and a younger disabled population. The needs of both populations are similar in severe disability, as is the impact of the disability. However, there are distinct differences between the support available, the expectations of the individuals compared to the younger population, and very often the aims of rehabilitation. The OPCS survey in 1988 showed that 32 per cent of people with disabilities living in private households were aged 75 years and over, 26 per cent were between the ages of 65 and 64 and 19 per cent between the ages of 55 and 64.

The question of survival following the acquisition of a physical disability is often asked when doctors prepare medical reports in cases of personal injury litigation. The risks for survival are fairly straightforward and the presence of epilepsy and the prevalence of recurrent chest and urinary infections are important in reducing life expectancy estimates. However, the most indicative in both adults and children is immobility, with all its attendant problems, which have been described earlier in the book. This whole issue can been studied further and the further reading list indicates where.

Further reading

Andrews, K. (1987). *Rehabilitation of the older adult*. Edward Arnold, London.

Barnes, M. P., Braithwaite, W., and Ward, A. B. (1997). *The medical aspects of personal injury litigation*. Blackwell Scientific, Oxford.

Calne, D. B., Comi, G., Crippa, D. *et al*. (1989). *Parkinsonism and ageing*. Raven Press, New York.

Index

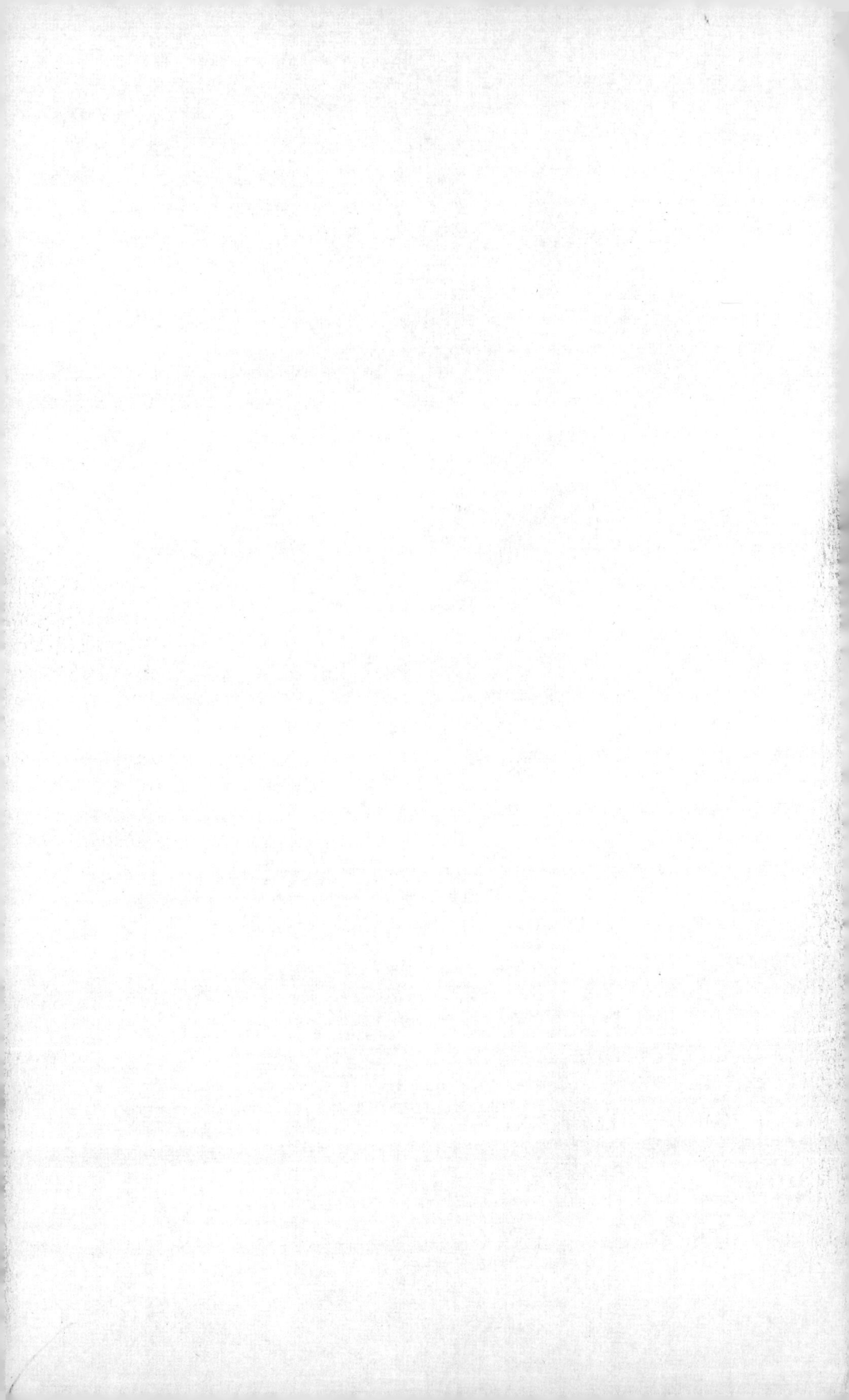